W9-BWX-299

Viral Hepatitis: Practical Evaluation and Treatment

Dedication

To my wife, Marilyn, whose computer skills, editing
and encouragement made this book a reality.

Viral Hepatitis: Practical Evaluation and Treatment

Teddy F. Bader, MD

Assistant Clinical Professor of Medicine
Division of Gastroenterology
University of Colorado Health Sciences Center

Colorado Permanente Medical Group
St. Joseph Hospital
Denver, Colorado

Hogrefe & Huber Publishers
Seattle • Toronto • Göttingen • Bern

Library of Congress Cataloging-in-Publication Data

Bader, Teddy F., 1953–
Viral Hepatitis: Practical Evaluation and Treatment / Teddy F. Bader
Library of Congress Cataloging-in-Publication Data is available via the
Library of Congress Marc Database under the
LC Catalog Card Number 94-077724

Canadian Cataloguing-in-Publication Data

Bader, Teddy F., 1953–
Viral hepatitis

Includes bibliographical references and index.
ISBN 0-88937-133-4

1. Hepatitis, Viral   I. Title.
RC848.H43B3   1996   616.3'623   C94-931867-1

ISBN 0-88937-133-4
Hogrefe & Huber Publishers, Seattle • Toronto • Göttingen • Bern
First edition 1995
Second edition 1997

© Copyright 1997 by Hogrefe & Huber Publishers
USA: P.O. Box 2487, Kirkland, WA 98083-2487,
Phone (206) 820-1500, Fax (206) 823-8324
CANADA: 12 Bruce Park Avenue, Toronto, Ontario M4P 2S3,
Phone (416) 482-6339
SWITZERLAND: Länggass-Straße 76, CH-3000 Bern 9,
Phone (031) 300-4500, Fax (031) 300-4590
GERMANY: Rohnsweg 25, D-37085 Göttingen,
Phone (0551) 49609-0, Fax (0551) 49609-88

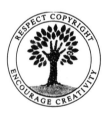

No part of this book may be reproduced, stored in a retrieval system, or
transmitted, in any form or by any means, electronic, mechanical, photo-
copying, microfilming, recording or otherwise, without the written permission
from the publisher.

Printed in USA

Acknowledgments

I wish to express my gratitude to those who have helped in writing this book. Dr. William Rector, Jr. was most gracious in reviewing Chapters 1–6 and 8–13 along with Chapter 15. His comments on style and substance greatly strengthened the text. Dr. Miriam Alter at the Centers for Disease Control reviewed Chapter 7 on the hepatitis B vaccine. Dr. Krzysztof Krawczynski, also at the Centers for Disease Control, reviewed Chapter 14 on hepatitis E. Dr. Paul Pinto and Dr. Phillip Steininger also furthered the project. Nikki Wilson Carroll performed the statistics in Chapter 9. Last, but not least, Dr. Robert Goo helped to co-author Chapter 12 and encouraged me to get started.

Foreword

Telfer B. Reynolds, M.D.
Clayton G. Loosli Professor of Medicine
University of Southern California
Los Angeles, California

Viral Hepatitis: Practical Evaluation and Treatment is an informative and "user friendly" text for health care workers on the front line. It is the first book on this subject area which has easy to find evaluation and treatment summaries. With numerous subheadings, one can read the text as a general overview or for as much detail as desired. It will allow primary care physicians to recognize and manage viral hepatitis in an efficient and up-to-date manner.

Unique aspects are: (1) the examination of disease outcome in both children and adults, (2) inclusion of material on hepatitis A vaccine, and (3) a discussion of the interaction of HIV disease with hepatitis B and C.

Dr. Bader has a long-term interest in viral hepatitis and sees it through the eyes of a physician who has witnessed the ravages of the disease in a high risk, poorly compliant segment of society—the prison population. Hence, his discussions of epidemiology and prevention are particularly well done.

The book is ideal for the busy clinician who will turn to it repeatedly for its easy access to relevant clinical information.

Foreword

Theodore C. Eickhoff, M.D.
Professor of Medicine
Division of Infectious Disease
University of Colorado School of Medicine

Here is a book whose title describes its content with absolute accuracy. It is a practical guide to the evaluation, diagnosis, treatment, and prevention of viral hepatitides from A through E. This volume should fill a great need for a single-source guide to viral hepatitis that will be welcomed by primary care physicians, including general internal medicine, family practitioners, and pediatricians as well. It is even possible, in this era of health care reform, to imagine a number of internal medicine subspecialists purchasing this volume as their own careers are redirected, at least in part, to primary care internal medicine.

The book is extraordinarily "user-friendly," a terribly over-used compound word that means only that the book is easily readable and well-indexed. It is very easy and quick to find one's way to a particular point of information that one wishes to know. Dr. Bader's style is simple and direct; there are no convoluted sentences or obfuscating phraseology. Perhaps best of all, there are summary outlines at the end of each chapter that will undoubtedly help to stimulate rapid recall. The text is richly supported by a large number of tables and graphs, and is well referenced for readers who wish to pursue particular points in greater depth.

So great has been the need for a practical and contemporary guide to viral hepatitis that in late 1993 the American Medical Association convened an expert Hepatitis Advisory Committee, and charged it with preparing a practical guideline for primary care physicians that will likely be very similar, albeit perhaps smaller in scope than this volume. Clearly, Dr. Bader has seen the need as well, and acted to fill it.

Finally, I must note for the record that it is a particular pleasure for me to write these words. Among the greatest rewards in academic medicine is to see one's students do well in their profession, and to make significant contributions to the nation's health. Dr. Bader, a former student of mine when I was his Internal Medicine Residency Program Director, has done exactly that. It was clear from the outset of his residency training that viral hepatitis was his first love in medicine, and it has remained so to this day. So committed was he to his goals in medicine that he served essentially two internships, one in family medicine, and one in internal medicine in order to achieve certification by the American Board of Internal Medicine in both Internal Medicine and Gastroenterology. My only wish is that I could have attracted Dr. Bader into my subspecialty of infectious diseases; it is clear, however, that he will have a distinguished career in gastroenterology.

Author's Preface

Viral hepatitis represents a fascinating set of diseases that cause a variety of symptoms and outcomes. I became interested in them as a medical officer for the United States Public Health Service in the federal prison system. Viral hepatitis often causes a total color change (jaundice) that usually subsides in a few weeks. When patients change color, it demands the attention of the patient, family and physician, to evaluate and treat the disease.

This book is written for a broad based audience of primary care providers such as those in internal medicine, family practice and pediatrics. The viewpoint is based in the United States, but an international perspective is also developed, since viral hepatitis is the most common chronic infectious disease in the world.

The material included is encyclopedic in breadth and covers most of the clinical problems likely to be encountered. At times, details are given on clinical problems which are of interest only if the problem is encountered. However, two editorial methods are used to help those attempting a general overview of the subject. First, numerous subheadings help the reader decide how far to delve into each topic. Secondly, some items are relegated to special topic chapters on hepatitis B and C.

An outline and summary of approach to each type of virus is at the end of every relevant chapter. This will allow the reader easy access to recall management issues.

In June 1996, an opportunity arose, because of a reprinting, to update and revise the book. New material has been added to chapters three, eight and twelve. These changes will make this revised edition effective for several more years.

All books are written from a particular bias and this one is no different. The author consistently attempts to develop a cost-effective approach to every problem. Testing is minimized. Immunization is preferred over any other form of therapy. Alfa-interferon 2b is preferred over liver transplantation. The natural history of chronic hepatitis B and C is emphasized, but many questions remain unanswered. The challenge to the clinician is to decide when to intervene with alfa-interferon 2b. All would agree that those patients with progressive liver disease should be treated. The trend is now to consider earlier treatment for those with minimal disease.

It is humbling to try to write a book such as this. I have become aware of a myriad of questions which exist. Despite my efforts and those of my reviewers, errors are doubtless present. The errors are all mine; I would be indebted to readers who bring them to my attention.

Medical References searched through PaperChase®.
PaperChase® is a registered trademark of Boston's Beth Israel Hospital.

Table of Contents

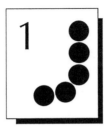

Overview of Viral Hepatitis

Approach to Diagnosis
General Therapeutic Measures

Approach to Diagnosis

At least five viruses are known to cause an organ specific infection of the liver referred to as viral hepatitis. Depending on a host of poorly understood factors, the infection may be entirely asymptomatic or deteriorate rapidly in a fulminant manner to death.

The focus of this chapter is to discuss the syndrome of viral hepatitis, present a brief overview of each virus along with diagnosis and general measures for treatment.

Hepatitis is defined as the presence of an elevated serum aminotransferase; in acute viral hepatitis, alanine (ALT) and aspartate (AST) aminotransferases often range from 1,000 to 3,000 IU/L (or more) with the ALT value higher than the AST. In chronic infections, the ALT value may be mildly elevated or even normal. The serum alkaline phosphatase is usually less than twice normal.

Only a minority of patients with acute or chronic viral hepatitis give a history of jaundice or any other classical symptom suggesting hepatitis. Patients may also report malaise, anorexia and influenza type symptoms. While a few symptoms may occur more commonly in one type of viral hepatitis than in another, the overlap is sufficient to state that no type of viral hepatitis can be reliably diagnosed on the clinical picture alone.

>> *There are no pathognomonic biochemical features of viral hepatitis. Clues to the diagnosis come from findings which support the presence of hepatocellular necrosis. Many other conditions cause a similar clinico-pathological picture and serological testing therefore becomes necessary.*

Health care professionals in every field encounter patients with acute or chronic viral hepatitis. Every physician and health care worker needs to understand three facts about each type of viral hepatitis: how to diagnose or classify viral hepatitis, modes of transmission, and whether the illness becomes chronic.

Hepatitis A

Hepatitis A is transmitted by fecal-oral means and does not cause chronic illness. It is diagnosed by the presence of IgM antibody in blood.

Hepatitis B

Hepatitis B is spread sexually and percutaneously (breakage of skin barriers with blood) and can lead to a chronic carrier state. It is diagnosed by the presence of an antigen called hepatitis B surface antigen. Occasionally, in acute illness, the patient will have already cleared HBsAg. For this reason, an IgM antibody to the core antigen is a superior test to diagnose the acute illness. Chronic hepatitis B is defined as the presence of HBsAg for more than 6 months.

Hepatitis C

Hepatitis C is spread percutaneously. Sexual transmission appears to occur very rarely or not at all. It is diagnosed by the presence of an IgG antibody to hepatitis C. The current second generation tests may only be 50% positive in the beginning of the acute illness and follow-up testing in 3 months is needed if the clinical picture warrants it. About 50% of patients infected with acute hepatitis C proceed to chronicity. As discussed in Chapter 10, the presence of a 12 month period of antibody to hepatitis C and abnormal aminotransferases is probably a better definition for chronic hepatitis C than the six month period often used.

Delta hepatitis

Delta hepatitis is spread in the identical manner as hepatitis B since it requires the hepatitis B surface antigen as an integral part of its virion structure. In other words, delta infection can only occur if the patient has concurrent hepatitis B. Chronicity often occurs and is defined in the same manner of six months as in hepatitis B. Delta hepatitis is diagnosed with either the IgM or IgG antibody. These antibodies are usually not present on most screening "viral hepatitis profiles." Total antibody to delta is usually present about 30 days after the onset of symptoms and in an acute case of hepatitis B, the delta antibody can be ordered at that time.

Hepatitis E

Hepatitis E is spread fecal-orally and produces a clinical picture similar to hepatitis A. The infection is not endemic in the United States. It occurs in Southeast Asia, India, Pakistan, Africa and Mexico.

A number of serological tests are in development but none are commercially available. If a patient has travelled recently to an endemic area and has unexplained hepatitis, testing can be pursued through the Centers for Disease Control, Atlanta, Georgia. Hepatitis E does not develop into a chronic infection.

Serology of viral hepatitis

The only serologic markers necessary in the first time evaluation of acute viral hepatitis are hepatitis A IgM, hepatitis B surface antigen, hepatitis B core antibody (IgM), and hepatitis C antibody (see Table 1.1).

Many laboratories hold specimens for testing of viral hepatitis and run tests once a week. While this weekly grouping may be cost-effective for the laboratory, it can result in a seven day delay in diagnosis. Since immunoprophylaxis is more effective the sooner it is given to contacts, clinicians need to be aware that specimens are collated for a run on a particular day of the week. If the day for serological testing has passed, the astute clinician can request a special run for the individual patient. Hospitals with an active blood bank perform daily assays for hepatitis B and C and a request for inclusion on the blood bank evaluation can also expedite results. The IgM HAV antibody is not part of the blood bank evaluation and is assayed separately. With this approach, results of testing for viral hepatitis return in 24 to 48 hours rather than the routine three to eight days.

Laboratories are beginning to automate the serology for viral hepatitis in the same manner as chemistry testing is performed. Automation should provide for daily analysis of viral hepatitis profiles and reduce the waiting time for diagnosis.

General Therapeutic Measures

Hospitalization is not necessary in most cases of viral hepatitis. However, viral hepatitis can rarely cause fulminant hepatitis (Chapter 15). By definition, fulminant hepatitis involves a change in mental status. Encephalopathy warrants hospitalization with aggressive management and the consultation of a liver specialist.

The prothrombin time is the best laboratory parameter that predicts severity of viral hepatitis. Should the prothrombin time be more than three seconds prolonged over control value, close observation is desirable.

Depending on the severity of the change in prothrombin time, a patient may be seen more frequently as an outpatient or even hospitalized. In conjunction with other variables listed in Table 15.2, a serum bilirubin greater than 17 mg/dl [300 µmol/L], can be a cause for concern.[1]

In contrast, the total bilirubin value does not predict severity of disease by itself and does not require hospitalization if the prothrombin time is normal.

Since the onset of fulminant hepatitis is usually in the seven to ten day range after symptoms begin,[2] it is wise to see an outpatient within seven days to be sure the mental status or prothrombin time is not deteriorating. Once a general improvement occurs, weekly visits are no longer necessary and follow-up to resolution or chronicity can take place with much longer monitoring intervals.

The degree of physical activity during acute, symptomatic cases does not affect the outcome of viral hepatitis. Repher's study of 398 servicemen with acute viral hepatitis randomly assigned to bedrest or vigorous one hour daily calisthenics and activity as desired, showed no difference in time to recovery or incidence of fulminant hepatitis.[3] However, the group assigned to strict bedrest experienced marked deconditioning resulting in a longer convalesence and a delay in return to work. Therefore, the patient should be off work and perform activity as desired while symptomatic.

Alcohol should be prohibited for six months (but preferably for one year) after acute viral hepatitis. Alcohol has been implicated in acute viral hepatitis progressing to fulminant hepatitis. It may also increase the possibility of the acute attack resulting in chronic hepatitis B, C or D. Alcohol also exacerbates the *post-hepatitis* syndrome. Prolonged fatigue, depression, etc. may persist after resolution of jaundice in any cause of viral hepatitis. This syndrome is seen in health care workers and military personnel and may be partly due to psychogenic causes.[4]

All non-essential medications should be discontinued. Oral contraceptives are safe to continue during acute viral hepatitis.[5]

Modern studies on the effect of major surgery during acute viral hepatitis are not available. Harville, in 1963, reported a 10% mortality and 12% major morbidity for laparotomy.[6] These complication rates are similar to other major operations for that period. Operative morbidity has declined significantly since 1970 and the above figures would likely be much better if studied again.[7] Nonetheless, patients with acute viral hepatitis should avoid elective surgery.

There is no proven dietary advice. Appetite is best in the morning and emphasis of caloric intake at that time of day is practical. Protein need not be restricted for fear of inducing encephalopathy; most observers suggest that the liver needs a high protein intake to regenerate optimally.

Finally, virtually every jurisdiction requires that cases of viral hepatitis be reported to the local health department.

Table 1.1 Diagnosing acute viral hepatitis.

	Anti-HAV IgM	HBsAg	Anti-HBc IgM	Anti-HCV
Acute hepatitis A	+	–	–	–
Acute hepatitis B	–	+	+	–
Chronic hepatitis B	–	+	–	–
Hepatitis C	–	–	–	+*

*As many as 50% of acute cases of hepatitis C tested by ELISA 2 may be sero-negative initially. If suspicion exists, repeat testing in three months is warranted.

Acute Viral Hepatitis Treatment Summary

1. Initiate rapid evaluation of serological results. Be aware of when the serological profile for viral hepatitis is being done in the local laboratory. If this is unsatisfactory, request special testing.
2. Evaluate patient for severity of disease.
   - Prothrombin time
   - Mental status
   - If prothrombin time and mental status are normal, patient may be followed as outpatient. First follow-up visit within seven days.
3. Prevent secondary cases.
   - Hepatitis A close contacts need immune serum globulin (Chapter 2).
   - Hepatitis B sexual contacts need HBIG and hepatitis B vaccine, if susceptible. Household members may need the vaccine (Chapter 7).
   - Hepatitis C—no proven prevention exists.
   - Delta hepatitis—same as for hepatitis B.
   - Hepatitis E—no proven prevention exists.
4. Make patient recommendations.
   - Activity and bedrest as desired. Patients will often require 4–6 weeks off work in order to recover. Time is variable.
   - Emphasize calories in a.m. since appetite is better.
   - Prohibit alcohol for one year.
   - Discontinue all meds possible until patient is well. (Oral contraceptives may be continued.)
   - Avoid elective surgery.
5. Hepatitis types B, C, and D need follow-up to determine if chronicity develops.
6. Report case to local health department.

References

1. O'Grady JG, Alexander GJ, Hayllor KM, et al. Early indicators of prognosis in fulminant hepatic failure. *Gastroenterology* 1989; 97:439–445.
2. Gimson A, White YS, Eddleston A, et al. Clinical and prognostic differences in fulminant hepatitis type A, B and non-A, non-B. *Gut* 1983; 24:1194–1198.

3. Repsher LH, Freebern RK. Effects of early and vigorous exercise on recovery from infectious hepatitis. *N Engl J Med* 1969; 281:1393–1396.
4. Sherlock S. *Diseases of the liver and biliary system.* Eighth edition. Oxford: Blackwell, 1989.
5. Schweilzer IL, Weiner JM, McPeak CM, et al. Oral contraceptives in acute viral hepatitis. *JAMA* 1975; 233:979–980.
6. Harville DD, Summerskill WH. Surgery in acute hepatitis. *JAMA* 1963; 184:257–261.
7. Bader T. Colorectal cancer in patients older than 75 years of age. *Dis Colon Rectum* 1986; 29:728–732.

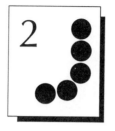

Hepatitis A

Clinical Manifestations

Hepatitis A (HAV) is an acute, self-limited disease caused by an RNA virus. HAV infection has a variable clinical course in which the symptom expression is markedly age dependent.

Table 2.1 lists symptoms that occur in children and adults. Most infections in children are asymptomatic compared to the low rate (16%) in adults. When children are symptomatic, the constellation of symptoms mimic an influenza type illness since jaundice is seldom overt in the young. Knowledge of the age related difference in symptom expression will help the clinician to discover sources of infection for the jaundiced adult. For example, the source may be a child who brought the infection home from a day care center either asymptomatically or with non-specific symptoms.

9

Table 2.1 Symptoms of hepatitis A in children and adults. Derived from references 1, 2, 3.

	Percent	
	Children	Adults
Nausea/vomiting	65	26
Jaundice/yellow eyes	65	88
Diarrhea	58	18
Abdominal pain	48	40
Malaise	48	63
Fever	41	18
Anorexia	41	40
Myalgia/arthralgia	6	30
Sore throat	6	0
Asymptomatic	73	16

Children are 2–5 years from day care epidemics and adults are from a military population.

The symptoms listed in Table 2.1 can describe any type of viral hepatitis. However, three features of HAV may provide clues to its presence: mildness of symptoms, jaundice and diarrhea. The mildness of the typical case of HAV is in contrast with the sicker patients with hepatitis B or C. This writer has heard a unique statement from young adults afflicted with HAV: "I am sorry to bother you doctor, since I feel well; but, my family wanted me to come see you since I have this yellow color to my skin." On a statistical basis, HAV is more likely to cause jaundice and/or diarrhea than the other hepatitis viruses. Fecal excretion of the virus may be responsible for diarrhea.[4](Figure 2.1)

The duration of jaundice in hepatitis A is usually seven to ten days (fig 2.2).[5] Besides jaundice, physical findings of HAV infection may be normal. Hepatomegaly and hepatic tenderness may occur in half of cases. Splenomegaly is less common. Ascites can occur.[6] Fever greater than 101°F (39°C) is not common in any form of viral hepatitis and its presence should cause the clinician to consider another diagnosis.

Laboratory findings include aminotransferase values that seldom exceed 1,000 IU. There is no correlation between the level of enzyme elevation and prognosis. Alkaline phosphatase is typically less than twice normal. Leukopenia is common and in 10% of cases the value is less than $5,000/mm^3$. Anemia and thrombocytopenia have been described but are much less common.[4]

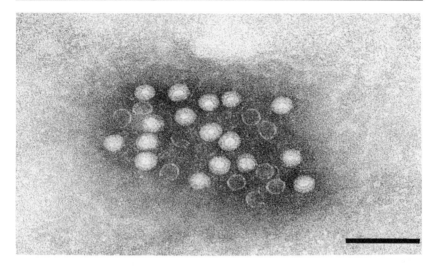

Figure 2.1 Electron micrograph of hepatitis A virus. From liver homogenates of infected marmosets. Complete and stain penetrated particles may be seen. Scale bar = 100 nm (×228,360). Photo courtesy of Dr. Hal Margolis and Dr. Charles Humphrey, CDC.

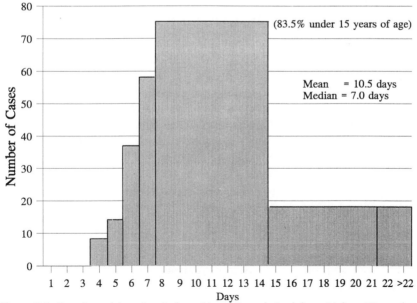

Figure 2.2 Duration of jaundice in hepatitis A. Data derived from Molaer JG, et al. Jaundice in Detroit. *Am J Public Health* 1940; 30:509.

The first signs of recovery are the disappearance of nausea and the return of appetite. The sense of well-being may improve despite the deepening of jaundice.[7]

With the onset of jaundice, symptoms such as arthralgias and myalgias abate. Anorexia and fatigue may worsen. Weight loss of 2–20 Kg is common.[7]

HAV is a disease manifested in young adults since more than 50% of cases occur in patients who are 20–39 years of age. The elderly (>75 years of age) in the United States have an immunity level of more than 80% making the chance of HAV in this group a remote possibility.

Uncommon Clinical Circumstances

Relapsing hepatitis A

Relapsing hepatitis A (RHA) is a condition in which resolution of symptoms and improvement in laboratory values occurs only to have a repetition of the clinical illness. The relapse takes place an average of four weeks after remission (range 1.5–18 weeks).[8] A relapse can occur more than once and HAV antigen is represent in the stool during relapse.[9] The incidence of RHA is in the 3.8–6.6% range. There are no predictive factors during the first illness that suggest relapse may occur and RHA does not prevent ultimate resolution.

Prolonged cholestasis

A significant number of uncomplicated cases will have jaundice lasting for a month. Rarely, *prolonged cholestasis*, jaundice lasting for two months or more can occur.[10]

Gordon and Schiff reported six cases of jaundice with the serum bilirubin levels of greater than 10 mg/dl (international value 170 µmol/l) lasting in the eight–twelve week range.[11] Clinical symptoms abate rapidly with a short course of oral prednisone.

Recognition of prolonged cholestasis due to hepatitis A is important in order to avoid studies such as endoscopic cholangiograms or exploratory laparotomy.[11]

Ultrasonic evaluation during HAV disease can be misleading in that thickening of the gallbladder wall occurs in both children and adults. Resolution of the thickening coincides with clinical resolution of HAV.[12]

Fulminant hepatitis A (see Chapter 15)

The frequency of fulminant hepatitis failure (FHF) in hepatitis A is extremely rare. It has been calculated as occurring in 0.14 and 0.35% of hospitalized cases in Australia and Greece, respectively. Since hospitalized cases represent a small minority of cases, the real prevalence of FHF in hepatitis A is considerably lower.[13] HAV is responsible for about 100 deaths annually in the United States. Refer to the treatment section later in this chapter, for management of FHF.

Extrahepatic manifestations

Hepatitis A, unlike hepatitis B, rarely has extrahepatic features. Two cases of arthritis, vasculitis with cryoglobulinemia have been reported.[14] One case of acalculous gangrenous cholecystitis[15], two cases of meningoencephalitis[4] and nine cases of acute oliguric renal failure are recorded.[16] Urticaria can also occur.[17]

Pregnancy

A report from Los Angeles lists six cases of hepatitis A occurring during pregnancy.[18] One developed during the second trimester and five during the third trimester. Five of the six women had complete recovery. One mother presented in the seventh month of pregnancy, delivered a premature infant, and died in fulminant hepatic failure two months later. Three mothers had acute hepatitis A at the time of delivery but anti-HAV was not detectable in the cord blood or the infant upon follow-up.

One case of vertical transmission of hepatitis A was recorded in a mother who became symptomatic ten days after delivering a premature infant. The infant became a source for an outbreak of hepatitis A in the neonatal intensive care unit.[19]

Glickson et al.[8] report a case in pregnancy where mild hepatitis A occurred in the first trimester and then the patient went into clinical remission for 18 weeks. The patient then relapsed with fulminant hepatitis and died. Interferon given during the relapse may have contributed to the poor outcome.

In developing countries, mortality during pregnancy with HAV has been significant. Nutrition must be the difference since, in developed countries, the pregnant woman with acute hepatitis A is felt to do no worse than her non-pregnant counterpart.[20, 21]

If immune serum globulin is needed during pregnancy, it is felt to be safe.[22]

Diagnosis

Acute illness due to hepatitis A is diagnosed by detection in serum of an IgM antibody to hepatitis A (Figure 2.3). The sensitivity of the IgM antibody is 100%; that is, there are no false negative results.[23] When patients are symptomatic, the IgM test will always be positive. The specificity of the IgM antibody is nearly perfect. Extensive testing of sera from conditions that might mimic hepatitis A found no false positive results (Table 2.2). The IgM antibody cut off value is designed to become negative 3 months after the onset of illness in most patients.[24] A few false positive IgM HAV cases have been noted without full documentation.[23] The IgM antibody can rarely be detected for as long as 18 months and persistence beyond this time should raise the suspicion of a false positive reaction.[25]

IgG antibody develops after the acute illness and represents immunity. Surveys of adults worldwide show an age-related prevalence of IgG antibody (Figure 2.3).

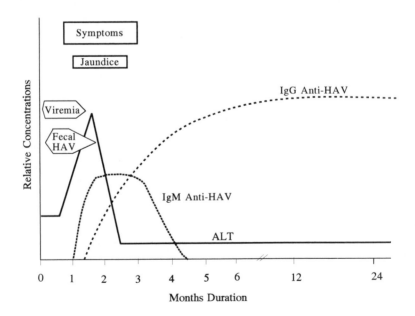

Figure 2.3 Clinical symptoms, viral presence and laboratory tests over a 24 month period.

Table 2.2 Reactivity of HAV IgM assay towards sera from normal subjects with other medical conditions. Used by permission. Decker RH, et al. Diagnosis of acute hepatitis A by HAVAB-M, a direct radioimmuno-assay for IgM anti-HAV. *Am J Clin Path* 1981; 76:146.

Specimens from:	Number tested	Number found positive
Acute rubella	9	0
Acute mononucleosis	22	0
Acute hepatitis B	9	0
Chronic hepatitis B	7	0
Alcoholic hepatitis	14	0
Rheumatoid factor	25	0
Anti-HAV IgG	14	0
Blood donors	100	0

Many laboratories hold specimens for testing of viral hepatitis and run the serological assay once a week. While this weekly run may be effective for the laboratory, it can mean as long as a seven day delay in obtaining results. Since immunoprophylaxis is more effective the sooner it is given to contacts, clinicians need to be aware that specimens are collated for a run on a particular day of the week. If the day for serological testing has passed, the effective clinician can request a special run for the individual patient. With this approach, results of testing for hepatitis A return in 24–48 hours rather than the routine seven days.

Infectivity

Inoculation studies have shown an incubation period ranging from 15 to 45 days with 28 days as an average. The principal mode of transmission is fecal-oral. HAV particles appear in the stool at least five days before the development of abnormal aminotransferase levels and jaundice. Fecal shedding of the virus is maximal in the late incubation period *before* the onset of symptoms and disappears about the time of maximal aminotransferase levels[27] (Figure 2.3). Experimentally induced infections cannot occur with body materials obtained four weeks before jaundice or more than 19 days after jaundice begins.[4]

A brief period of viremia lasting less than seven days and in very low concentration occurs in the late incubation period. As a result, transfusion associated HAV can rarely happen.[28]

Low levels of HAV antigen are present in urine, saliva and respiratory secretions. For salivary and respiratory secretions, the HAV present may only represent blood contamination. In any case, these body fluids are probably not important for transmission.[4]

Survival studies of HAV placed on the hands of human volunteers show a 20% residual amount of virus still existing on fingerpads after 4 hours. Transferrance of HAV from an inanimate surface to the human hand can occur up to 3 hours after placement on the surface.[29]

Data does not exist to determine the risk of heterosexual contact since studies do not distinguish close family contact from sexual involvement.

Epidemiology

Epidemics of hepatitis A can cause both economic and societal havoc. In the public's mind, hepatitis A infections are most commonly linked with restaurant associated outbreaks. However, this source accounts for only a small fraction of the total (Figure 2.3). Epidemics are associated with day care centers, military personnel and sporadic cases in travelers.

Asymptomatic food handlers can start epidemics of HAV that alarm an entire city; suspected restaurants suffer economic havoc which may result in their closing.

>> *A food handler for a large catering business in Denver, Colorado transmitted hepatitis A to 43 patrons of office parties during a recent holiday season. Thousands of fearful patrons deluged their physicians' offices to receive the temporary (three month) protection afforded by gamma globulin injection. Restaurant business in general diminished for a while and the popular caterer barely avoided bankruptcy and reopened the business 60 days later.*

Many types of food have been reported to become contaminated with sewage infected with hepatitis A. With the exception of shellfish, the contamination is probably passive. Raw clams are a frequent cause of epidemics. Steaming the clam does not appear to provide a high

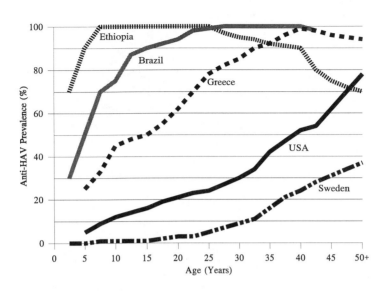

Figure 2.4 Patterns of HAV seroprevalence worldwide: I—very low, II—low, III–intermediate, IV—high, V—very high. Figure in Public Domain (reference 26).

enough temperature to kill the virus.[30–32] Food handlers are also sources of epidemics.[4]

Day care centers cause a large number of hepatitis A cases (Figure 2.4). Reports have ranged from 14 to 40% of cases in the United States, depending on the population studied.[33, 34] The risk factor appears to be diaper changing with fecal-oral contamination. However, HAV contamination of toys and other items may persist for prolonged periods of time.[29] The child is often asymptomatic but brings his infection home to his parents who then develop symptoms without suspicion of their origin.

Hepatitis A has been a major problem throughout history for military campaigns. Epidemics of hepatitis A reached staggering proportions in the Second World War: 200,000 cases occurred among U. S. troops and 5,000,000 cases occurred among German armies and civilians alone. American soldiers with acute hepatitis missed six to eight weeks of duty.[35, 36]

Squalid conditions and close contact also led to major problems in refugee and prisoner of war camps. Indeed, the number of cases was so significant as to influence the strategy of the war.[36]

The negative impact on troops caused the British and U.S. armies to authorize a series of studies among human volunteers to define the

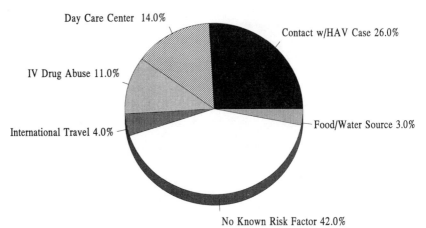

Day Care Center 14.0%

Contact w/HAV Case 26.0%

IV Drug Abuse 11.0%

International Travel 4.0%

Food/Water Source 3.0%

No Known Risk Factor 42.0%

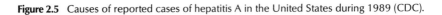

Figure 2.5 Causes of reported cases of hepatitis A in the United States during 1989 (CDC).

basic features of the disease and to devise methods for its control.[37] Prior to these studies, it was not fully accepted that viral hepatitis was an infectious disease.

HAV infections are increasing among homosexual men. A 1991 survey from the Centers for Disease Control of Denver, New York City, San Francisco, Toronto, Montreal and Australia revealed that in young men presenting with HAV disease, 42 to 78% are homosexual.[38] The predisposition for HAV disease in homosexuals probably reflects fecal-oral contamination.

Data from the CDC also show an increasing association between drug abuse and hepatitis A in the United States.[39] Between 1982 and 1986, the percentage of persons with hepatitis A who admitted to previous IV drug use rose steadily from 4% to 19%. Also, IV drug abusers have a much higher prevalence of HAV IgG antibodies.

While it is possible that HAV may be transmitted by injection, it seems more likely that the drugs are being contaminated with fecal material at the cultivation site or direct person to person transfer is occurring under poor hygenic conditions common to drug abusers.[39]

Travelers from developed countries are often exposed and become ill during visits to endemic areas (Figure 2.5). The incidence of clinical hepatitis A developing among European tourists visiting endemic areas and staying only in good quality accommodations is estimated to be between three and six per 1,000 per month. If the tourist backpacks, the incidence is thought to be 20 per 1,000 per month.[37]

Prevalence of Infection

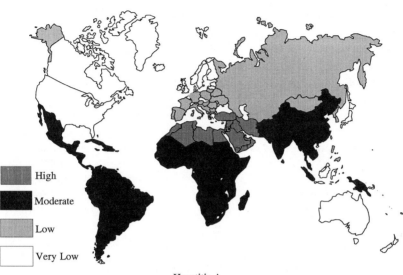

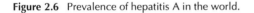

Hepatitis A

Figure 2.6 Prevalence of hepatitis A in the world.

Two common vehicles of transmission then represent the usual source of infection: close contact with an HAV infected person or contact with contaminated sewage. Most transmission occurs before the onset of symptoms and attempts to quarantine active cases do little to forestall epidemics.[40]

Prevention

Travel (pre-exposure prophylaxis)

The risk of acquiring HAV when traveling abroad varies with living conditions, length of stay and incidence of HAV in the area. Travel to western Europe, Canada, Japan, Australia and New Zealand provides no greater risk than in the United States. High risk areas for HAV exposure are the middle East, Southeast Asia, Africa, Central and South America and eastern Europe[22, 41] (Figure 2.5).

Visiting rural areas or planned contact with children increases the risk. However, a recent study showed hepatitis A occurring in travelers to developing countries who had "standard" tourist itineraries, accommodations and food.[22]

In addition to ISG prophylaxis, travelers should avoid water and ice of unknown purity. Boiling water (98°C) for one minute inactivates HAV.[42] The consumption of food should follow the *rule of three P's*: a *packaged* source, *piping* hot or *peeled* by the traveler himself.

If travelers are frequent visitors to endemic areas, it is useful to check their serum IgG level for HAV immunity. Since immunity correlates with age, a cost-effective decision may be to only check travelers above age 35 for presence of the IgG antibody.[41] If the IgG antibody is positive, no ISG prophylaxis is necessary. The other way to avoid repetitive ISG doses is to receive the hepatitis A vaccine now available in Europe (see Chapter 3). It is hoped the hepatitis A vaccine will be released soon in the United States. Avoiding what can be a painful gluteal ISG shot before sitting on a long, transcontinental flight becomes an item of great appreciation to the veteran traveler.

Post-exposure prophylaxis (Tables 2.3 and 2.4)

Immune serum globulin (ISG) administered to close contacts within two weeks of exposure has a 90% protective rate. Dose-response studies show that 0.02 ml/kg is the optimal level.[43] The dose for short term travel is identical to that for postexposure prophylaxis.

The administration of ISG does not result in serum antibody levels detectable by available immunoassay methods.[1] Thus, in cases of acute hepatitis A occurring despite ISG administration, usual serodiagnostic criteria apply.

Safety of immune globulins

Immune globulins made in the United States have few side effects. The primary side effect is soreness at the injection site. ISG does not transmit hepatitis B, C or the HIV virus.[22] The cost of ISG is not a concern. 1.0 cc of ISG is about $2.

Treatment

Treatment of HAV disease involves evaluating the severity of disease, advice on hygienic measures and prevention of secondary cases. The evaluation of severity of disease is reviewed in Chapter 1. The patient with HAV is almost non-infectious upon presentation with symptoms. Fecal shedding of the virus has usually stopped or will do so in a few

Table 2.3 Recommendations for immune globulin post-exposure prophylaxis for hepatitis A (CDC, reference 44).

Close personal contact	All household and sexual contacts of persons with HAV.
Day-care centers	Staff, attendees, and all members of households whose diapered children attend.
Common-source exposure	Not warranted once cases have begun to appear, since the 2-week period during which ISG is effective will have been exceeded. When a food handler with HAV is identified, ISG should be given to other food-handlers and may be considered for patrons if:
	a. the infected person is directly involved in handling foods that are not to be cooked or cooked foods before they are eaten
	b. the hygiene practices of the worker are deficient *and*
	c. patrons can be identified and treated within two weeks of exposure.
Institutions for custodial care	Depending on the circumstances, prophylaxis may be limited or can involve the entire institution.
Hospitals	Routine ISG use is not indicated. In outbreaks, prophylaxis of persons exposed to feces of infected patients is indicated.
Schools, offices and factories	Casual contact in these situations does not result in virus transmission and ISG is not indicated.

days. Therefore, sexual partners should avoid intimate contact for one week after the onset of illness. A one week abstinence with the 90% protection rate provided by ISG will make sexual contraction of HAV unusual.

Commercial food handlers, day care workers and health care workers should be off work for at least one week after symptoms begin and for as long as symptoms (especially diarrhea) persist. Many adult workers will require one to four weeks off work. Complete resolution of jaundice is not required before returning to work except in food handlers or those workers who have a significant social interaction. Customers at a restaurant or other places of business may shy away from employees who are jaundiced for fear of a contagious disease. The decision to return to work should depend on how the patient feels, not necessarily on liver function tests. Counsel about fastidious hygiene and careful handwashing after use of the toilet is essential.

Table 2.4 Immune globulin for protection against viral hepatitis A (reference 22.)

Length of stay	Body weight		Dose volume*	Comments
	lb	*kg****		
Short-term travel	<50	<23	0.5 ml	Dose volume
(<3 mos)	50–100	23–45	1.0 ml	depends on body weight & length
Post-exposure prophylaxis	>100	>45	2.0 ml	
Long-term travel	<22	<10	0.5 ml	
(>3 mos)	<50	<23	1.0 ml	
	50–100	23–45	2.5 ml	
	>100	>45	5.0 ml	

*For intramuscular injection   **1 kg = approximately 2.2 lbs

Relapsing and prolonged cholestasis

Reports of small numbers of patients treated with cortiocosteroids have shown prompt improvement in both of these conditions.[8,11] A long taper of the corticosteroid is needed to prevent recurrence of cholestasis.[11]

Fulminant hepatitis A

Survival for FHF caused by hepatitis A and treated medically in a special liver unit is 80%.[13] The one year survival rates for liver transplantation in acute liver failure ranges from 55 to 75%.[13] Thus, it is vital to properly select the small proportion of patients who will need a new liver (Chapter 15).

The new liver graft appears to often become reinfected with hepatitis A and a symptomatic episode can occur. HAV antigens can be demonstrated as long as seven months after transplantation.[47] Ultimate clearance of the hepatitis A virus from the new graft should occur.

Acute Hepatitis A Treatment Summary

1. Hepatitis A IgM antibody is diagnostic of acute disease. HAV IgG antibody indicates remote infection and current immunity.
2. Evaluate patient for severity of disease.
   - Prothrombin time.
   - Mental status.
   - If prothrombin time and mental status are normal, patient may be followed as outpatient. First follow-up visit within seven days.
3. Prevent secondary cases.
   - Close contacts need immune serum globulin in a dose of 0.02 ml/kg. A body weight table is shown in Table 2.4. Other risk groups are defined in Figure 2.7.
   - Avoid sexual relations for one week.
4. Patient recommendations:
   - Activity and bedrest as desired.
   - Emphasize calories in a.m. since appetite is better then.
   - Prohibit alcohol for one year.
   - Discontinue all meds possible until patient is well.
   - Avoid elective surgery.
   - Meticulous washing of hands after passage of feces.
   - Jaundice lasts seven to ten days in most cases.
5. Report case to local health department.

References

1. Lemon SM. Type A viral hepatitis: new developments in an old disease. *N Engl J Med* 1985; 313:1059–1067.
2. Lednar WM, Lemon SM, Kirkpatrick JW. Frequency of illness associated with epidemic hepatitis A virus infections in adults. *Am J Epidemiol* 1985; 122:226–233.
3. Benenson MW, Takafuji ET, Bancroft WH, et al. A military community outbreak of hepatitis type A related to transmission in a child care facility. *Am J Epidemiol* 1980; 112:471–481.
4. Zakin D, Boyer TD, eds. *Hepatology: a textbook of liver disease.* Philadelphia: W. B. Saunders, 1990.
5. Molner JG, Meyer KF. Jaundice in Detroit. *Am J Public Health* 1940; 30:509–515.
6. Dagan R, Yagupsky P, Barki Y. Acute ascites accompanying hepatitis A infection in a child. *Infection* 1988; 16:360–361.

7. Hoofnagle JH. Acute viral hepatitis clinical features, laboratory findings, and treatment. In: Berk JE, Haubrich WS, Kalser MH, eds. *Bockus gastroenterology.* Philadelphia: W.B. Saunders, 1985.

8. Glickson M, Galun E, Oren R, et al. Relapsing hepatitis A: review of 14 cases and literature survey. *Medicine* 1992; 71:14–23.

9. Sjogren MH, Tanno H, Fay O, et al. Hepatitis A virus in stool during clinical relapse. *Ann Intern Med* 1987; 106:221–226.

10. Gimson A, White YS, Eddleston A, et al. Clinical and prognostic differences in fulminant hepatitis type A, B and non-A, non-B. *Gut* 1983; 24:1194–1198.

11. Gordon SC, Reddy KR, Schiff L, et al. Prolonged intrahepatic cholestasis secondary to acute hepatitis A. *Ann Intern Med* 1984; 101:635–637.

12. Foulner D. Sonographic gallbladder wall thickening in children: association with acute hepatitis A. *Australas Radiol* 1991; 35:333–335.

13. O'Grady J. Management of acute and fulminant hepatitis A. *Vaccine* 1992; 10 (suppl 1): S21–26.

14. Inman RD, Hodge M, Johnston M, et al. Arthritis, vasculitis and cryoglobulinemia associated with relapsing hepatitis A virus infection. *Ann Intern Med* 1986; 105:700–703.

15. Black MM, Mann NP. Gangrenous cholecystitis due to hepatitis A infection. *J Trop Med Hygiene* 1992; 95(1):73–74.

16. Geltner D, Naot Y, Zimhoni O, et al. Acute oliguric renal failure complicating type A non-fulminant viral hepatitis. *J Clin Gastroenterol* 1992; 14:160–162.

17. Scully LJ, Ryan AE. Urticaria and acute hepatitis infection. *Am J Gastroenterol* 1993; 88:277–278.

18. Tong MJ, Thurshy M, Rakela J, et al. Studies on the maternal-infant transmission of the viruses which cause acute hepatitis. *Gastroenterology* 1981; 80:999–1004.

19. Watson JC, Fleming DW, Borella AJ, et al. Vertical transmission of hepatitis A resulting in outbreak in a neonatal intensive care unit. *J Infect Dis* 1993; 167:567–571.

20. Seeff LB. Viral Hepatitis and prenancy. In: Rustgi VK, Cooper JN, eds. *Gastrointestinal and hepatic complications in pregnancy.* New York: John Wiley, 1986: 179–199.

21. Wilkinson ML. Diagnosis and management of liver disease in pregnancy. *Adv Intern Med* 1990; 35:289–310.

22. U.S. Dept. of Health and Human Services. *Health information for international travel 1990.* Washington, D.C.: U.S. Government Printing Office, 1990.

23. Hoofnagle JH. Serologic diagnosis of acute and chronic hepatitis. *American Association for Study of Liver Diseases.* Presentation October 29, 1989. Program pages 187–190.

24. Decker RH, Kosakowski SM, Vanderbilt AS, et al. Diagnosis of acute hepatitis A by HAVAB-M, a direct radioimmuno-assay for IgM anti-HAV. *Am J Clin Pathol* 1981; 76:140–147.

25. Kao HW, Ashcavai M, Redeker A. The persistence of hepatitis A IgM antibody after acute clinical hepatitis A. *Hepatology* 1984; 4:933–936.

26. Hadler SC. Global impact of hepatitis A virus infection changing patterns. In: Hollinger FB, Lemon SM, Margolis H, eds. *Viral hepatitis and liver disease: proceedings of the 1990 International Symposium on viral hepatitis and liver disease: contemporary issues and future prospects.* Baltimore: Williams and Wilkins, 1991:14–20.

27. Dienstag JL, Feinstone SM, Kapikian AZ, et al. Fecal shedding of hepatitis A antigen. *Lancet* 1975; 1:765–767.

28. Hollinger FB, Khan NC, Oefinger PE, et al. Posttransfusion hepatitis type A. *JAMA* 1983; 250:2313–2317.

29. Mbithi JN, Springthorpe S, Boulet JR, et al. Survival of hepatitis A virus on human hands and its transfer on contact with animate and inanimate surfaces. *J Clin Microbiol* 1992; 30:757–763.

30. Portnoy BL, Mackowiak PA, Caraway CT, et al. Oyster-associated hepatitis. *JAMA* 1975; 233:1065–1068.

31. Sherlock S. *Diseases of the liver and biliary system.* Eighth edition. Oxford: Blackwell, 1989.

32. Desenclos JA, Klontz KC, Wilder MH, et al. A multistate outbreak of hepatitis A caused by the consumption of raw oysters. *Am J Public Health* 1991; 81:1268-72.

33. Shapiro CN, Coleman PJ, McQuillan GM, et al. Epidemiology of hepatitis A: seroepidemiology and risk groups in the USA. *Vaccine* 1992; 10 (Suppl 1):S59–62.

34. Hadler SC, Webster HM, Erben JJ, et al. Hepatitis A in day-care centers. *N Engl J Med* 1980; 302:1222–1227.

35. Bancroft WH, Lemon SM. Hepatitis A from the military perspective. In: Gerety RJ, ed. *Hepatitis A.* Orlando: Academic Press, 1984:81–100.

36. Hoke CH, Binn LN, Egan JE, et al. Hepatitis A in the US army: epidemiology and vaccine development. *Vaccine* 1992; 10 (Suppl 1):S75–80.

37. Gust ID. A vaccine against hepatitis A—at last. *Med J Aust* 1992; 157:345–346.

38. Centers for Disease Control. Hepatitis A among homosexual men—United States, Canada, and Australia. *MMWR* 1992; 41:155–164.
39. Centers for Disease Control. Hepatitis A among drug users. *MMWR* 1988; 37:297–300.
40. Rakela J, Mosley JW. Fecal excretion of hepatitis A virus in humans. *J Infect Dis* 1977; 135:933–938.
41. Kendall BJ, Cooksley WE. Prophylactic treatment regimens for the prevention of hepatitis A. *Drugs* 1991; 41:883–888.
42. Krugman S, Giles JP, Hammond J. Hepatitis virus: effect of heat on the infectivity and antigenicity of the MS-1 and MS-2 strains. *J Infect Dis* 1970; 122:432–436.
43. Masterson RG, Strike PW, Teltmar RE. Hepatitis A immunity and travel history. *J Infection* 1991; 23:321–326.
44. Centers for Disease Control. Protection against viral hepatitis: recommendations of the immunization practices advisory committee. *MMWR* 1990; 39: number S-2.
45. Winokur PL, Stapleton JT. Immunoglobulin prophylaxis for hepatitis A. *Clin Inf Dis* 1992; 14:580–586.
46. Shapiro CN. Transmission of hepatitis viruses. *Ann Intern Med* 1994; 120:82–84.
47. Fagan E, Yousef G, Brahm J, et al. Persistence of hepatitis A virus in fulminant hepatitis and after liver transplantation. *J Med Virol* 1990; 30:131–136.

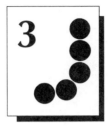

Hepatitis A Vaccine

Production
Safety
Immunogenicity
Pre-Exposure Efficacy
Post-Exposure Efficacy
High-Risk Groups
Children
Combined Active and Passive Immunization
Simultaneous Vaccination Against Hepatitis A and B
Pre and Post Antibody Testing

Hepatitis A (HAV) is a universal infection with immunity acquired during childhood in developing countries of the world. A contrasting pattern of infrequent exposure to HAV exists in developed nations. In countries with good sanitation, less than 10% of the population develops HAV antibody by age 20 (Chapter 2, Figure 2.3). Usually asymptomatic in children, hepatitis A can cause severe disease as susceptible contacts become older; the increasing lack of immunity towards HAV in the United States portends a greater disease burden in the future.

While hepatitis A does not evolve into chronic infection and cause cirrhosis, epidemics cause significant temporary disability in individuals and havoc to society.

The titer of hepatitis A antibody is diminishing in gamma globulin (ISG) preparations since these lots are drawn from the general population. The decreasing effectiveness of gamma globulin along with the temporary protection ISG affords (2–3 months), leads to the distinct need for a safe and effective hepatitis A vaccine.

HAV should be easily preventable with a vaccine since there is a single viral serotype and no significant antigenic variation.

Production

The hepatitis A vaccine currently approved in many parts of Europe, Havrix® (SmithKline Beecham Biologicals, Rixensart, Belgium), is made in an extensively monitored and purified manner.

An approach similar to development of inactivated polio vaccines is used for the inactivated hepatitis A vaccine (Figure 3.1). An HAV strain (HM 175) is injected into a normal, human diploid cell line known as MRC-5. The virus multiples in these cells and is then separated, inactivated and standardized. The cell line used is free of extraneous agents, shows normal karyology and lacks tumorigenicity. It has been used for more than 20 years in the production of vaccines such as rubella, measles and mumps; it has a good record of safety.[1] The adjuvant, aluminum hydroxide, has been used in inactivated vaccines for more than 30 years.[2]

Once the vaccine process was established, it was shown to be safe and effective in animal studies. Phase I, II and III trials in humans have also shown the vaccine to be highly immunogenic and effective.[3]

A similar inactivated vaccine is being tested by Merck, Sharpe and Dohme (MSD). An HAV strain, CR 326F, is also inoculated into MRC-5 cells and produced in a like manner.[4] The MSD vaccine has not yet been approved for clinical use in any country.

Early attempts in the 1980's focused on a live, attenuated HAV vaccine. The attenuated viruses appear to replicate poorly in their human hosts and thus generate a weak immune response. In addition, attenuated HAV strains cause a transient, low-level elevation of aminotransferases. The greatest hope for the live vaccine was that it could be given orally; but, infectivity or immunogenicity does not occur with attenuated strains given orally.[3, 5]

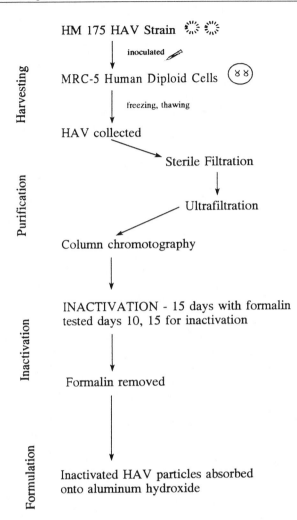

Figure 3.1 Production of an inactivated hepatitis A vaccine (Havrix®). Data derived from Peetermans J. Production, quality control and characterization of an inactivated hepatitis A vaccine. *Vaccine* 1992; 10 (Suppl):S99–101.

The remainder of this chapter will focus on the killed virus vaccine, Havrix®, which has the most research and clinical information yet reported.

Safety

More than 1,000,000 doses of inactivated hepatitis A vaccine have been given worldwide. Side-effects have been mild and of no importance. Soreness or transient redness at the injection site is reported with 34 to 44% of inoculations.[6, 7] This effect is shared by all alum-adjuvant vaccines. Other general symptoms reported are less than 10% (Table 3.1) and represent the same profile of symptoms with the administration of placebo.[8]

A trend towards decreased frequency of both local and general signs has been noted after successive doses of the vaccine.[9] This indicates there is no induction of clinical hypersensitivity to the vaccine.

Immunogenicity

Antibody levels induced by vaccine or gamma globulin require a more sensitive assay than the standard commercial immunoassays such as the Havab assay (Abbott Laboratories, North Chicago, IL) measure. Sensitivity of the standard Havab assay may be enhanced 10-fold by

Table 3.1 General and local adverse reactions following Havrix® injection in adults. Andre PE, et al. Clinical assessment of the safety and efficacy of an inactivated hepatitis A vaccine: rationale and summary of findings. *Vaccine* 1992; 10 (Suppl 1): S160–168. By permission of the publishers, Butterworth Heineman Ltd©.

Symptom	Proportion of doses (%) leading to reported symptom
General symptoms	
Fever	4.0
Headache	8.9
Malaise	5.7
Loss of appetite	1.9
Nausea	3.2
Vomitimg	0.5
Fatigue	9.1
Local symptoms	
Soreness	34.7
Induration	7.8
Redness	5.9
Swelling	9.1

increasing the volume of serum tested by a factor of ten. The "modified Havab" test is capable of detecting anti-HAV at a level of approximately 10 mIU/ml and will detect antibody levels given by gamma globulin which are known to be protective.[7]

>> *Antibody levels in the following discussion are derived from modified assays and are not available from the clinician's usual laboratory.*

The standard dose of Havrix® vaccine for adults in the United States is 1440 ELISA units in 1 cc of solution. In clinical studies involving over 400 healthy adult volunteers, a single dose of 1440 ELISA units elicited seroconversion (defined as ≥ 20 mIU/ml) in more than 96% of subjects at one month. By day 15, 80–98% of vaccinees had responded. Geometric mean titers (GMT) of responders ranged from 264 to 339 mIU/ml at day 15 and increased to a range of 335 to 637 mIU/ml by one month (Figure 3.3).[10] With a primary dose of 1440 ELISA units, antibody levels will be measurable for one to two years. With a booster dose at 6–12 months, it is estimated that antibody levels will be detectable for at least six to seven years.[11] Whether immunity extends beyond detectable antibody levels, as with hepatitis B vaccination, remains to be determined.

The adult formation of the hepatitis A vaccine in many countries outside the United States contains 720 ELISA units per cc dose. This lower concentration vaccine series consists of a primary dose at 0 and 1 month and a booster dose at 12 months. This three dose regimen also achieves 100% seroconversion with similar antibody levels to the two dose series in the United States. The makers of the vaccine, Smith Kline and Beecham, eventually plan to have every country use the two dose (1440 ELISA) series for adults.

Primary immunization (i.e. 1440 ELISA unit dose or two doses of 720 ELISA units at 0 and 30 days) should provide protection in fourteen days after its completion.[10]

Pre-Exposure Efficacy

Chimpanzees vaccinated with Havrix® and then challenged with virulent HAV do not become ill in contrast to non-vaccinated cohorts.[12]

A large vaccination trial is available from Thailand, an endemic area for HAV, where over 40,000 young volunteers received either Havrix® or hepatitis B vaccine as placebo. The first dose was given January, 1991. At the conclusion of the study, 40 cases of symptomatic HAV infection were reported, with 38 occurring in placebo recipients. The protective efficacy was 95%. The two infections which took place in vaccine recipients occurred after only two doses and were very mild with only slight increases in alanine aminotransferase.[13]

A placebo-controlled trial, in 1,037 children from a community in New York which experienced periodic outbreaks of HAV, was performed with a similarly inactivated HAV vaccine by Merck, Sharpe and Dohme. Before adequate immunity developed by day 21, seven cases occurred in the vaccine group and three cases in the placebo group. However, after day 21, 34 cases occurred in the placebo group and none in the vaccine group for an efficacy rate of 100%.[14]

Thus, in the pre-exposure setting, the inactivated hepatitis A vaccine clearly prevents HAV infection both in direct challenge studies and in large, placebo controlled trials.

Post-Exposure Efficacy

Little work has been done concerning post-exposure vaccination to prevent hepatitis A. Two chimpanzees were given a gastric inoculation of hepatitis A and vaccinated (720 ELISA units) 1 and 3 days after exposure. One chimpanzee had no evidence of infection, while the other developed a mild ALT elevation. Neither of the animals had detectable fecal excretion of HAV RNA. In the same study, 2 control chimpanzees developed typical cases of hepatitis A with detectable fecal excretion of HAV.[15]

In a marmoset study,[16] seven animals were challenged with HAV and then four were vaccinated 48 hours later with a 360 ELISA unit dose and three were given a 1440 ELISA unit dose. Three of four marmosets receiving the lower dose of vaccine developed hepatitis A. However, viral excretion in the feces was reduced in quantity and duration compared to controls. All three animals receiving the larger 1440 unit dose were completely protected from developing hepatitis A.

In comparison, ISG administered to post-exposure human contacts within two weeks of exposure has a 90% protection rate (chapter two). The effect of ISG on fecal excretion of HAV is unknown.[15] More work needs to be done before the hepatitis A vaccine can be considered as a replacement of ISG in the post-exposure setting.

High-Risk Groups

Figure 3.2 outlines groups at particular risk of acquiring hepatitis A and members of these groups are candidates for receiving the vaccine.

Universal vaccination, an eventual long-term goal, will probably not be promoted at the current time. The only reason for this limitation is cost. Safety and efficacy are not issues. The cost of Havrix® is comparable to the hepatitis B vaccine at about $40 per dose.

The first seven groups in Figure 3.4 have been commented on extensively in Chapter 2. A few additional comments will be made here.

Vaccination of food handlers will stop many but not all epidemics associated with food. Food can become passively contaminated with HAV by being sprayed or washed with contaminated water. Shellfish, particularly oysters, can actively take up the HAV virus from contaminated ocean water.

The presence of intravenous drug abusers (IVDA) listed in Figure 3.2 may seem incongruous to the reader. HAV is only rarely spread through percutaneous routes since the period of viremia is less than 24 hours. It is thought that occurrence of HAV in this situation results from the unsanitary conditions associated with IVDA rather than the use of needles.[17]

Day-care Center Child/Attendant

Military Personnel

Food Handler

Travel to Endemic Area

Contact with HAV Case

Male Homosexuals

Sewage Worker

Intravenous Drug Abuse

Health Care Worker

Closed Institution Occupants

Figure 3.2 High-risk groups for acquiring or spreading hepatitis A.

Certain types of health care workers (HCW) are at risk of contracting HAV. The hazard appears related to the degree of stool exposure. Thus, nurses and cleaning personnel are at higher risk than physicians.[18-20]

Closed institutions, such as those for the mentally disabled, represent a well-documented arena for outbreaks of HAV.[20-21]

Community epidemics are difficult to stop with immune serum globulin (ISG). Infections may occur in two or three cycles and the temporary protection afforded by ISG disappears. Vaccination is the logical approach to eliminate smoldering epidemics of HAV.[21]

Children

The worldwide pediatric formulation of the hepatitis A vaccine has a concentration of 360 ELISA units for a one cc dose. Three doses are recommended in a 0, 1, and 6 to 12 month schedule. Using this schedule, 100% of children above one year of age seroconvert with antibody levels nearly identical to those achieved in adults.[10,22] One study noted good antibody responses in children from three months of age to six years of age.[23] There is a concern that maternally derived antibody to HAV may interfere with the vaccine response in newborns of seropositive mothers.[24] The hepatitis A vaccine has been approved for use in children two years of age and older in the United States.[10] As of April 1, 1996 a new pediatric dose was approved by U.S. Food and Drug Administration. The approved formulation is a 720 ELISA unit injection in two doses rather than three. The second is given 6–12 months after the first.

Combined Active and Passive Immunization

Investigators in Belgium examined the effect of combining immune serum globulin (ISG) with the inactivated hepatitis A vaccine given into different injection sites. ISG was given in a large dose of 5 ml; this is about 0.04 ml/kg or twice the usual prevention dose. As noted in Figure 3.3, the administration of ISG causes immediate antibody levels at day five but lessens the antibody levels achieved at seven months by nearly 50%.[25] The attenuation of vaccine effect by ISG in hepatitis A is in contrast to hepatitis B where HBIG does not interfere with the efficacy of the hepatitis B vaccine.

The combination of ISG and hepatitis A vaccine offers the advantage of immediate protection but at the disadvantage of lowering ultimate antibody levels. Further work is needed to examine the interaction of these modalities. Perhaps delaying the timing of the first dose of vaccine to one or two months after the ISG would improve final antibody levels.

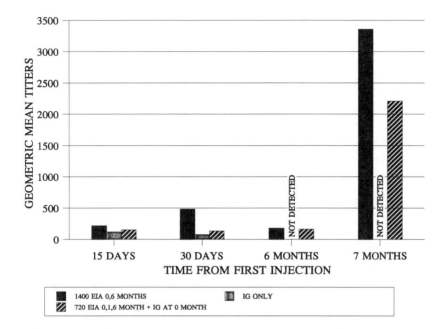

Figure 3.3 Geometric mean titers of antibody for hepatitis A with 1400 EIA dose alone, immune globulin alone, and vaccine + immune globulin. The three dose 720 EIA and two dose 1400 EIA vaccines give quite similar antibody levels at serum months (3,967 vs. 3,360, respectively). No data available for IG combined with 1400 EIA dose. Data combined from references 25, 30, 31.

Simultaneous Vaccination Against Hepatitis A and B

The simultaneous administration of hepatitis A vaccine (Havrix®) and hepatitis B vaccine (Engerix B®) into separate muscle areas in young adults causes the same antibody levels to both hepatitis A and B as when given alone.[26] Side-effects of this approach are no different.

Another study, of a German produced inactivated hepatitis A vaccine given at the same time with Engerix-B, also showed no interference of the vaccines; in fact, the antibody level to hepatitis A was significantly higher at twelve weeks in the combined group as compared to the group receiving hepatitis A vaccine alone.[27]

Pre and Post Antibody Testing

Post-vaccination testing for hepatitis A antibody is not necessary since 100% of adults and children above two years of age seroconvert.

Pre-testing for IgG antibody to HAV is only cost-effective if the patient has a suggestive history of prior exposure or possesses certain demographic features. If a patient reports a prior history of "hepatitis," this is likely to be a hepatitis A event. Also, if the patient grew up in an endemic country or is above age 40, antibody screening is likely to be cost-effective. Based on experience with hepatitis B immunization, a pre-test probability of greater than 20% prevalence of HAV antibody existing in a population should be present before testing.[28]

Antibodies to HAV are quite age-dependent. A local study of antibody rates at the author's institution shows that testing prospective vaccine candidates above age 40 to be cost-effective.[29]

Further work needs to be done in this area and each country will need to delineate their local demographics to maximize health care expenditures.

Summary

A drastic decline in disease related to hepatitis A has occurred in the 20th century due to improvements in sewage control and sanitation. Curtailment of HAV in developed countries is a mixed blessing in that subsequent birth cohorts have not developed immunity and few young adults are naturally protected; an asymptomatic disease, universal in children due to poor sanitation, has been converted into a less frequent but much more symptomatic disease in adults. Obviously, for a number of health reasons, a return to poorer sanitation levels is not a solution.

Immune serum globulin (ISG) has helped reduce the number of cases resulting from direct contact. However, only temporary defense (three months) is offered without permanent protection. In post-exposure situations, ISG must be given within seven days of exposure, necessitating costly and impracticable disease surveillance for early case detection. ISG is rarely used effectively in the post-exposure setting due to the need of swift prophylaxis. The large doses of ISG and repeated administration needed for pre-exposure travel prophylaxis make it a painful and costly approach to hepatitis A prevention.

The currently available hepatitis A vaccine surmounts all the difficulties associated with ISG use in a safe and effective manner. High-risk groups will certainly benefit from the use of the hepatitis A vaccine. However, as has been learned from the hepatitis B vaccine, universal vaccination will eventually be needed to greatly reduce the impact of this disease on society.

References

1. Peetermans J. Production, quality control and characterization of an inactivated hepatitis A vaccine. *Vaccine* 1992; 10 (Suppl 1):S99–101.

2. Shapiro CN, Coleman PJ, McQuillan GM, et al. Epidemiology of hepatitis A: seroepidemiology and risk groups in the USA. *Vaccine* 1992; 10-(Suppl 1):S59–62.

3. Hadler SC, Webster HM, Erben JJ, et al. Hepatitis A in day-care centers. *N Engl J Med* 1980; 302:1222–1227.

4. Hoke CH, Binn LN, Egan JE, et al. Hepatitis A in the US army: epidemiology and vaccine development. *Vaccine* 1992; 10 (Suppl 1):S75–80.

5. Gust ID. A vaccine against hepatitis A—at last. *Med J Aust* 1992; 157:345–346.

6. Lewis JA, Armstrong ME, Larson VM, et al. Use of a live, attenuated hepatitis A vaccine to prepare a highly purified, formalin-inactivated hepatitis A vaccine. In: Hollinger FB, Lemon SM, Margolis H, eds. *Viral hepatitis and liver disease: proceedings of the 1990 Internationl Symposium on Viral Hepatitis and Liver Disease.* Baltimore: Williams and Wilkins, 1991:94–97.

7. Tilzey AJ, Palmer SJ, Barrow S, et al. Clinical trial with inactivated hepatitis A vaccine and recommendations for its use. *Br Med J* 1992; 304:1272–1276.

8. Andre FE, D'Hondt E, Delem A, et al. Clinical assessment of the safety and efficacy of an inactivated hepatitis A vaccine: rationale and summary of findings. *Vaccine* 1992; 10 (Suppl 1):S160–168.

9. Lemon SM. Inactivated hepatitis A virus vaccines. *Hepatology* 1992; 15:1194–1197.

10. Product insert. Hepatitis A Vaccine. Smith, Kline and Beecham. Philadelphia, Pennsylvania, USA

11. Wiedermann G, Ambrosch F, Andre FE, et al. Persistence of vaccine-induced antibody to hepatitis A virus. *Vaccine* 1992; 10 (Suppl 1):S129–131.

12. Purcell RH, Hondt ED, Bradbury R, et al. Inactivated hepatitis A vaccine: active and passive immunoprophylaxis in chimpanzees. *Vaccine* 1992; 10 (Suppl 1):S148–151.

13. Innis BL, Snitbham R, Kunasol P, et al. Protection against hepatitis A by an inactivated vaccine. *JAMA* 1994; 271:1328–1334.

14. Werzberger A, Mensch B, Kuter B, et al. A controlled trial of a formalin-inactivated hepatitis A vaccine in healthy children. *N Engl J Med* 1992; 317:453–457.

15. Robertson BH, D'Hondt EH, Spelbring J, et al. Effect of post-exposure vaccination in a chimpanzee model of hepatitis A virus infection. *J Med Virol* 1994; 43:249–51.

16. D'Hondt E, Purcell RH, Emerson SU, et al. Efficacy of an inactivated hepatitis A vaccine in pre- and postexposure conditions in Marmosets. *J Infect Dis* 1994; 171 (Suppl 1):S40–3.

17. Centers for Disease Control. Hepatitis A among drug users. *MMWR* 1988; 37:297–300.

18. Longson PJ. Hepatitis A Vaccine. *Br Med J* 1992;305: 888.

19. Hofmann F, Wehrle G, Berthold H, et al. Hepatitis A as an occupational hazard. *Vaccine* 1992; 10 (Suppl 1):S82–84.

20. Rajan E, Albloushi S, Farrell BO, et al. Nurses in a general adult hospital are also at increased risk of hepatitis A infection. *Am J Gastroenterology* 1993; 88:1555A (abstract).

21. Prospects for control of hepatitis A: panel discussion. *Vaccine* 1992; 10 (Suppl 1):S170–174.

22. Lee SD, Lo KJ, Chan CY, et al. Immunogenicity of inactivated hepatitis A vaccine in children. *Gastroenterology* 1993; 104:1129–1132.

23. Horng YC, Chang MH, Lee CY, et al. Safety and immunogenicity of hepatitis A vaccine in healthy children. *Pediatr Infect Dis J* 1993; 12:35–62.

24. Lemon SM, Shapiro CN. The value of immunization against hepatitis A. *Infect Agents and Disease* 1994; 1:38–49.

25. Leentvaar-Kuijpers A, Coutinho RA, Brulein V, et al. Simultaneous passive and active immunization against hepatitis A. *Vaccine* 1992; 10 (Suppl 1):S138–141.

26. Ambrosch F, Andre FE, Delem A, et al. Simultaneous vaccination against hepatitis A and B: results of a controlled study. *Vaccine* 1992; 10 (Suppl 1):S142–145.

27. Flehmig B, Heinricy U, Pfisterer M. Simultaneous vaccination for hepatitis A and B. *J Infect Dis* 1990; 161:865–868.

28. Hashimoto F. Cost-effectiveness of serotesting before hepatitis vaccination. *N Engl J Med* 1982; 307:503.

29. Bader TF. Hepatitis A vaccine. *Am J Gastroenterology* 1996; 91: 217–22.

30. Briem H, Safary A. Immunogenicity and safety in adults of hepatitis A virus vaccine administered as a single dose with a booster 6 months later. *J Med Virology* 1994; 44:443–5.

31. Victor J, Knudsen JD, Nielsen LP, et al. Hepatitis A vaccine. A new convenient single-dose schedule with booster when long-term immunization is warranted. *Vaccine* 1994; 12:1327–9.

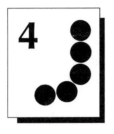

Acute Hepatitis B

Hepatitis B is the most common chronic infectious disease in the world. Over 300 million people worldwide are infected with the virus. While most chronic carriers reside in Asia and Africa, 1.5 million are thought to reside in the United States. 300,000 acute infections with HBV occur each year in the United States.[1] The magnitude of the HBV problem warrants the concern and complete understanding of every health care worker.

Baruch Blumberg discovered hepatitis B serindipitously in 1964 while searching for genetic markers in population groups. A distinct protein found by electrophoresis was consistently noted in sera of Australian aborigines. Further observations associated the protein, named *Australian antigen*, with viral hepatitis. *Hepatitis associated antigen* became the new name of the virus as it was quickly utilized as a screening test for blood donors in 1969. Discovery of the hepatitis A virus in stool and development of serology in 1973 led to the hepatitis associated antigen being renamed hepatitis B surface antigen. Dr. Blumberg received the Nobel prize in 1977 for his discovery. For a description of the discovery and early issues surrounding hepatitis B, the interested reader is referred to reference two.

The literature of HBV is voluminous and growing. Over 800 articles a year are published in English on MEDLINE concerning clinical studies in humans beings alone! In an effort to avoid a reference list running over a thousand items, only the latest or most comprehensive article will be cited. The reader can then obtain the citation and additional sources.

The Virus

Hepatitis B is a unique virus containing both double stranded and single stranded DNA. The intact Dane particle and surface antigen particles are portrayed in Figure 4.1. Figure 4.2 illustrates the component parts of the virus. The clinician needs to master the basic terminology in order to understand the stages of hepatitis B. The following section generalizes about the serology of HBV. Unusual profiles are discussed in Chapter 6 on *Difficult Serology*.

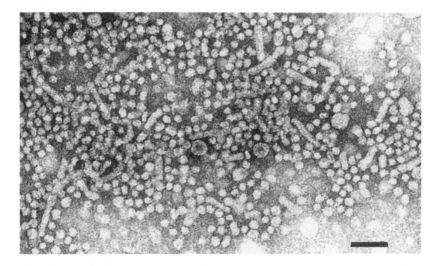

Figure 4.1 Electron microscopy of hepatitis B virus in negatively stained human serum. Spherical 42 nm Dane (intact virion) particles, 22 nm HBsAg, and filamentous particles are present. Scale bar = 100 nm (×118,800). Photo courtesy Dr. Hal Margolis and Dr. Charles Humphrey, CDC.

Structure of HBV

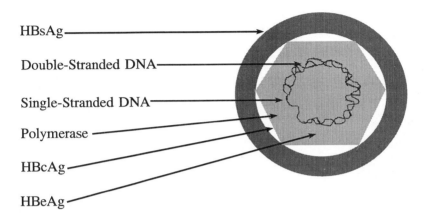

HBsAg

Double-Stranded DNA

Single-Stranded DNA

Polymerase

HBcAg

HBeAg

Figure 4.2   Schematic structure of hepatitis B virus.

The hepatitis B surface antigen (HBsAg) is an incomplete, non-replicating part of the virus that for unknown reasons is produced in large quantity by the virus. As many as 10^{15} surface antigen particles may exist in the bloodstream and by weight in some carriers this may exceed the albumin level!

Antibody to the surface antigen is called surface antibody (anti-Hbs). It appears in resolving infections two to three months after symptoms begin. Anti-Hbs represents convalescence and immunity. Anti-Hbs and HBsAg are generally exclusive of each other.

The Dane particle, or complete virion, is present in much smaller quantity than the surface antigen. It has an interior core antigen (HBcAg) which is detected in liver tissue but not in blood; thus, there is no serological test for it. Antibody to the core antigen is referred to as the core antibody and appears together in both the IgM class (acute disease) and IgG class (convalescent or chronic infection). The core antibodies coexist with either HBsAg or anti-Hbs depending on the stage of HBV infection. The core antibody does not confer immunity.

Another marker, the hepatitis "e" antigen (HBeAg), is a subparticle of the core antigen. It appears in acute infection simultaneously with the surface antigen and generally reflects viral replication. The antibody to HBeAg (anti-Hbe) denotes that viral replication has stopped or is at a very low level. Anti-Hbe does not confer immunity. The "e" marker system is *not* needed to diagnose acute or chronic hepatitis B.

This writer finds that the "e" markers confuse many practitioners and the discussion of its role will be limited to the specific topics of infectivity and chronic hepatitis B.

Acute Hepatitis B

In the United States, the majority of acute infections from HBV occur in young adults and teenagers. In this age group, 50% of infections are asymptomatic; another 30% are subclinical, and only 20% are overtly ill with jaundice and severe symptoms.[3] A subclinical infection has symptoms similar to influenza and will not be diagnosed as acute hepatitis unless blood is drawn for liver function tests. A common misunderstanding by those unfamiliar with the field of viral hepatitis is to equate acute or chronic hepatitis B with jaundice. Only a small proportion of patients with acute or chronic HBV infection give a history of jaundice. Furthermore, since jaundice is much more common in hepatitis A, a prior undocumented history of icterus will usually relate to an illness caused by hepatitis A rather than hepatitis B. It is not understood why some patients develop jaundice and others do not. Anicteric patients tend to have fewer symptoms and a lower mortality rate but may be more likely to advance to a chronic carrier state.

Studies of the prevalence of symptoms in acute viral hepatitis were published prior to the introduction of serology for hepatitis and thus represent *contaminated* data representing 4 or more viruses. The best clinical data on acute HBV infection comes from two sources: (1) the epidemic caused by the yellow fever vaccine during World War II; and, (2) the National Institutes of Health inoculation studies on federal prisoners performed in the years 1951 to 1954. Both of these groups have subsequently been shown by retrospective serology to have been clearly infected by the hepatitis B virus.[4,5,6]

The yellow fever vaccine, given to U.S. Army personnel in 1942, caused an epidemic of jaundice. The jaundice occurred an average of 14–15 weeks after vaccine administration. The vaccine had been stabilized with human serum contaminated with hepatitis B virus. Vaccine administration was stopped but over 50,000 U.S. Army personnel were affected before the epidemic subsided. Prevalence of symptoms (Table 4.1) and medical conditions (Table 4.2) were studied in 398 cases.[7]

The list of symptoms for hepatitis B in Table 4.1 are similar in degree to those listed in Table 2.1. As a result, one cannot reliably diagnose the type of viral hepatitis by symptoms alone. However, there are a number of features which may suggest that the patient with *acute viral*

Table 4.1 Incidence of symptoms (%) in icteric hepatitis B. Series I—soldiers infected during WWII. Series II—experimental transmission cases 1951–1954. Derived from Hayman JM, et al. Some clinical observations on an outbreak of jaundice following yellow fever vaccination. *Am J Med Sci* 1945; 209:281-300 and Barker LF, et al. Acquistion of hepatitis-associated antigen. *JAMA* 1971; 216:1970-6.

	Series I	Series II
Anorexia	79	79
Nausea	65	75
Weakness	51	NA
Epigastric discomfort	46	NA
Vomiting	34	46
Diarrhea	12	NA
Malaise	10	79
RUQ pain	7	70
Urticaria	3	NA

hepatitis has hepatitis B. Severity of illness, longer prodromal period and extrahepatic symptoms can provide clues to the presence of HBV.

While comparative disability studies have not been done, it seems that patients with acute hepatitis B are much less able to perform

Table 4.2 Incidence of physical findings (%) in icteric hepatitis B. Series I—398 soldiers in WWII. Series II—experimental transmission cases 1951–1954. Derived from Hayman JM, et al. Some clinical observations on an outbreak of jaundice following yellow fever vaccination. *Am J Med Sci* 1945; 209:281-300 and Barker LF, et al. Acquisition of hepatitis-associated antigen. *JAMA* 1971; 216:1970-6.

	Series I	Series II
Hepatomegaly	72	51
Liver tenderness	53	76
Palpable spleen	7	NA
Maximum temperature		
<99°F (37°C)	85	NA
<101°F (38.3°C)	14.5	NA
<104°F (40°C)	0.5	NA

activities of daily living and require more bedrest than those afflicted with acute hepatitis A or C.

Uncommon Clinical Features of Acute Hepatitis B

The prodromal period is longer in hepatitis B with a mean period of 7 days compared to 60% of patients with hepatitis A who have symptoms for one day or less.[8] A serum sickness-like or arthritis-dermatitis syndrome is the most common prodrome occurring in the late incubation period of hepatitis B (i.e. before jaundice appears). Retrospective studies have shown an incidence of arthritis symptoms ranging from 1 to 49%.[6] The arthritis is often symmetric and involves the small joints of the hands as commonly as the knees. In descending order of frequency, wrists, ankles, elbows, shoulders and hips can also be involved.[9]

The arthritic symptoms may resolve when jaundice begins or may continue or appear at the time of initiation of jaundice. Arthritis can occur without jaundice. The arthritis usually resolves in three to seven days but three cases of continuous arthritis with persistent HBV infection have been noted. No deformity or joint destruction occurs. Table 4.3 provides a comparison of HBV related arthritis and rheumatoid arthritis.

Dermatologic manifestations are varied and occur in a minority of patients.[11, 12] Urticaria is most common and can be the only presenting complaint. Angioedema, palpable purpura, erythema nodosum,

Table 4.3 Comparison between rheumatoid and HBsAg positive arthritidies. Derived from McCarty DJ, et al. Arthritis and HBAg-positive hepatitis. *Arch Int Med* 1973; 1321:216-8.

	Rheumatoid Arthritis	HBsAg Positive Arthritis
Symmetric, polyarticular arthritis	+	+
Morning stiffness	+	+
Synovial thickening	+	−
Rash	−	−
Fever, increased ESR	+	−
HBsAg	−	+
Rheumatoid factor	+	−
Joint deformity and destruction	+	−

erythema multiform and lichen planus may also develop. Skin manifestations can occur in anicteric cases and in the absence of arthritis.

Neurologic manifestations are uncommon. Seizures are rare in acute hepatitis B.[13] Encephalomyeloradiculitis (Guillain-Barré syndrome) has been documented in eight cases of hepatitis B. The CSF contained HBsAg in those studies and all patients recovered with little deficit. Polyneuritis is usually manifested as a peripheral neuropathy but cranial nerve involvement does occur.[14] Nerve conduction velocities have been shown to be impaired even in the absence of neurological symptoms and resolve as the disease subsides.[15] Mononeuritis multiplex, an asymmetric sensorimotor neuropathy, occurs in HBsAg positive periarteritis nodosa.

Patients with hepatitis B rarely manifest important cardiac disease. Myocarditis, pericarditis and arrythmias occur, usually in the setting of fulminant hepatitis, and may contribute to the cause of death.[14, 16]

Pleural effusion is the only pulmonary abnormality that is attributed to HBV. Effusions are rare and when examined usually contain HBsAg and HBeAg. The effusions can occur in both overt and anicteric hepatitis B.[14]

Acute pancreatitis commonly occurs in fulminant hepatitis but its involvement in uncomplicated hepatitis B is uncertain.[17] Elevated pancreatic isoenzymes and radiological evidence supporting pancreatitis have been reported.[18] While the preceding reports are from a time period prior to HBsAg testing it is likely they represent predominantly, if not solely, HBV disease. The pancreas may be an important non-hepatic site of HBV replication. HBsAg has been shown by immunofluorescence techniques in the pancreas of 18 out of 30 infected persons. Core antigen (replicating form) was detected in six of the patients.[19] Further evidence supporting the association of HBV and pancreatitis comes from the observation that pancreatitis is a peculiar event following liver transplantation for hepatitis B. Alexander, et al, report hyperamylasemia in 6 of 27 patients and 4/27 with clinical pancreatitis post-transplantation for HBV compared to none of their control group.[20]

Mild proteinuria and slight abnormalities of urinary sediment may occur in icteric patients. Red cells and red cell casts can be noted.[21] These sediment changes exist independent of the membranous glomerulopathy that occurs in chronic hepatitis B. Renal failure apart from fulminant hepatitis and chronic HBV is rare. Patients can have either a functional pre-renal type picture or acute tubular necrosis. Patients with renal failure but without fulminant hepatitis recover completely unless sepsis intervenes.[22] Aplastic anemia can occur in hepatitis B.[14]

Laboratory Findings

Laboratory abnormalities include aminotransferase levels ranging from 1,000 to 4,000 IU/liter.[23] Total bilirubin levels seldom exceed ten mg/dl (340 μmol/L) in icteric cases. After peaking, bilirubin usually declines by 50% per week. Bilirubin values greater than 30 mg/dl (510 μmol/L) signify hemolysis or renal failure. The hemolysis associated with sickle cell anemia or glucose-6-phosphate dehydrogenase deficiency can cause marked hyperbilirubinemia when viral hepatitis occurs in these patients.[14]

Laboratory tests which may cause confusion over the etiology of the liver disease include elevated serum iron and copper levels.[14] To the unwary, these values may suggest hemochromatosis or Wilson's disease particularly in the setting of fulminant hepatitis where the patient with HBV disease may be seronegative for HBsAg.

Alpha fetoprotein (AFP) levels are elevated in acute viral hepatitis[24] and appear to correlate with a good prognosis.[25] It is thought that AFP is a sign of liver regeneration in viral hepatitis but not all authors agree. AFP measured during the acute or convalescent phase of hepatitis B could mislead the clinician into needless concern about hepatocellular carcinoma complicating the case.

Diagnosis of Acute Infection

The serological phases of acute infection in icteric patients are depicted in Figures 4.3 and 4.4. It is reemphasized that jaundice occurs in a minority of cases (20% or fewer) of infected individuals.

The incubation period from time of exposure to symptoms is 100 days[7] (range 28–225 days).[21] HBsAg appears in the serum as early as one or two weeks and as late as 11 or 12 weeks after exposure to HBV.[6, 26] The form of inoculation exposure and the laboratory detection method determines the time of appearance of HBsAg. Testing by complement fixation (an insensitive test) detects the surface antigen 29–43 days after parenteral exposure and 67–82 days after oral exposure. With the highly sensitive radioimmunoassay, HBsAg can be detected as early as six days after parenteral exposure. Symptoms occur about four weeks (range 3–6) after the appearance of HBsAg in the blood.[6, 26]

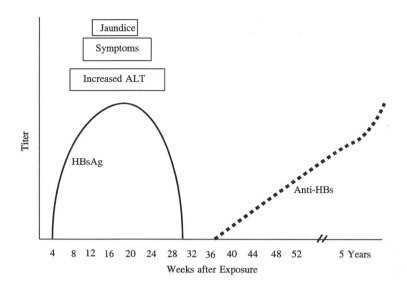

Figure 4.3 HBV infection with resolution of surface antigen-antibody system.

As symptoms resolve, the titer of HBsAg falls and becomes undetectable several weeks after the biochemical hepatitis normalizes.
However, in experimental studies, 9% of patients are surface antigen

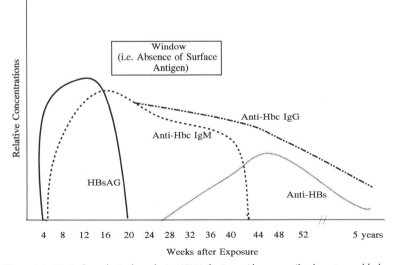

Figure 4.4 Typical serological results in HBV infection with core antibody system added.

negative before the onset of symptoms and 28% clear HBsAg at the time of symptom resolution.[26]

Antibody to surface antigen usually appears one to three months after the disappearance of HBsAg. The antibody titer rises slowly during recovery for up to 12 months.[26] In the 10 to 20% fraction of patients who experience prodromal HBV arthritis and rash, anti-Hbs appears at the same time as the HBsAg and together with HBsAg forms immune complexes.[27] Another 10% of patients will never form measurable anti-Hbs and will have only anti-Hbc as evidence of disease exposure. It is not understood why these individuals do not form surface antibody, but they are immune from second infections with HBV.[6]

Antibodies to the core antigen can be detected about four weeks after HBsAg begins and these antibodies always appear before clinically apparent hepatitis. Anti-Hbc consisting of both IgM and IgG arises during the period of HBsAg positivity. After HBsAg disappears, the IgM anti-Hbc falls off much more rapidly than IgG but in up to 20% of patients it can persist for two years.[27] Anti-Hbc of the IgG class drops after its initial peak but falls very slowly. IgG anti-Hbc persists for many years[26] and lasts longer than surface antibody. The anti-HBc marker system would not be utilized except that as many as 12% to 46% of patients who present with clinical hepatitis due to acute HBV will be surface antigen negative.[6, 28] Since there is a gap of several months between HBsAg and its antibody, these patients would be seronegative for HBV disease. This gap is referred to as the *window* period. During the window period, anti-Hbc of either the IgG or IgM class will be present (Figure 4.4). Anti-HBc of the IgM class indicates acute HBV infection. Depending on the level of viral replication, some chronic carriers may also have low titers of IgM anti-Hbc present.

To summarize, typical results on an acute hepatitis B viral profile are shown in Table 4.4.

Liver biopsy is not indicated in uncomplicated acute hepatitis B with documented HBsAg of less than six months duration. The reason

Table 4.4 Typical serological results in HBV infection.

HBsAg	Anti-HBc IgM	Anti-HBs	Interpretation
+	+	−	Acute HBV infection
−	+	−	Acute HBV infection
+	−	−	Chronic HBV infection
−	−	+	Prior HBV infection or vaccination

for not performing a liver biopsy is that the histology is misleading and a weak predictor of outcome.[29]

Liver biopsy may be indicated in the *persistent* (i.e., lasting four months) hepatitis B case that appears to be declining clinically since the discovery of *bridging necrosis* may predict the development of chronic liver disease in as many as one third of cases.[14, 30] If bridging necrosis is not found, all patients recover. Ware, et al, in a retrospective study found that one of 57 patients with bridging necrosis (two-thirds of whom were HBsAg positive) died and eight developed chronic liver disease. However, the patient that died received corticosteroids.[31] Overall, most patients with subacute hepatic necrosis (see next section) recover completely.[30]

Natural History of Acute Hepatitis B

Serological profiles illustrated in Figures 4.3 and 4.4 fail to demonstrate the wide biological variation inherent in any disease. When symptoms or jaundice persist for two or three months, undue worry can develop that an *unusual* case is present. The point at which a *typical* case becomes *prolonged* is entirely arbitrary. The duration of acute hepatitis is known to vary with a host of factors mentioned below. Four months is the time limit beyond which adults would usually be considered to have a *prolonged course* of hepatitis B.[30]

In resolving cases, HBsAg can disappear any time over four months after symptoms appear (Figure 4.5). In most cases, HBsAg persists until symptoms or biochemical abnormalities resolve but in some patients the reverse is true. The median time of HBsAg clearance is seven weeks after symptoms begin. The severity of the hepatitis, as measured by the degree of bilirubin elevation, roughly correlates with the duration of HBsAg positivity.[6]

In a small group (<3%), HBV disease worsens over a period of one to three months. In this entity, *subacute hepatic necrosis*, jaundice deepens and a gradual deterioration of coagulation factors occurs. Signs suggestive of the development of portal hypertension such as ascites, peripheral edema and splenomegaly appear. Features that correlate with the occurrence of subacute hepatic necrosis are the development of HBV in persons older than 40 years of age, drug addiction and the insidious onset of anicteric disease.[14]

The least common outcome of acute HBV disease is *fulminant hepatitis*. This term is applied when hepatic failure and encephalopathy occur abruptly in the first eight weeks of illness. The incidence of

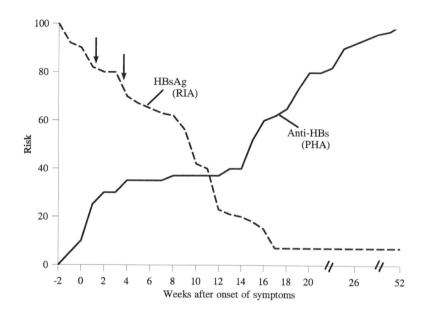

Figure 4.5 The percent of patients positive for HBsAg and anti-HBs by week after onset of symptoms. Used by permission of J. Hoofnagle. Figure in Public Domain.

fulminant hepatitis occurs in less than 1% of HBV cases. Fulminant hepatitis is discussed more fully in Chapter 15.

Development of a chronic carrier state, defined as HBsAg positivity for more than six months, can occur in 1%–95% of cases depending on a number of factors. Important determinants are: (1) age of the individual when infected; (2) gender; (3) the form of expression of the acute disease; and (4) the immune status of the infected host.[32]

The greatest influence on the development of chronicity is age of the individual at the time of infection (Figure 4.3). 90% of neonates, 20% of children and 1–5% of adults infected will become chronic carriers (Figure 4.6). Infected males have a 1.6× likelihood of becoming a carrier compared to females.[33] Furthermore, the mean annual clearance rate of HBsAg in female carriers is 1.9% compared to 0.4% for males.[34] Chronic HBsAg development occurs more frequently in anicteric cases than in icteric hepatitis.[35]

The differences that immune status can cause is best illustrated from HBV infection in dialysis units. Dialysis patients have a mild illness and a chronic carrier rate of 40 to 90%[27]; whereas, dialysis staff develop icteric hepatitis that resolves completely in almost all instances.[32] Other immune deficiency states which have increased incidence of develop-

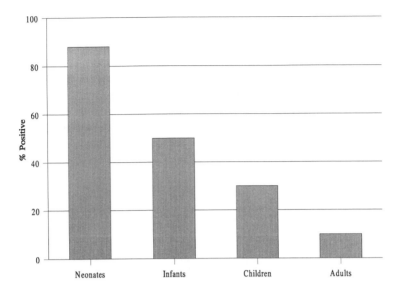

Figure 4.6 Risk of carrier state after acute infection versus age. Adapted with permission from Unit 3, Viral Hepatitis, A Clinical Teaching Project of the American Gastroenterological Association.

ing chronic HBV infection are hemophilia, HIV disease and individuals with Down's syndrome.[8]

Whether race or ethnic origin predisposes to a chronic carrier state is not clear.[32] Blacks and Oriental populations have a higher rate of chronic hepatitis B than the Caucasian population.[36] From population studies, Blumberg suggests that susceptibility to persistent infection is inherited as an autosomal recessive trait.[2]

It is widely taught that 5–10% of patients with acute hepatitis B advance to the HBsAg carrier state. Given the above data on influencing factors, the 5–10% figure should not be taught at all; instead, a notation of the fact should be made that chronicity varies widely depending upon a number of defined and undefined factors.[36]

Figure 4.7 summarizes the possible outcome of acute HBV disease in adults. Figure 4.8 illustrates the effect of age on symptomatic expression and chronic carrier rate.

Infectivity

The hepatitis B virus is a hardy agent capable of withstanding wide extremes of temperatures and chemical agents. It remains stable after

Acute Hepatitis B in Adults

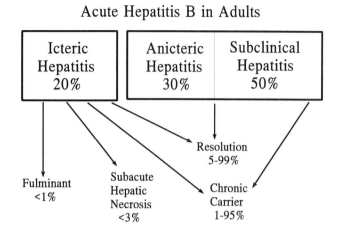

Figure 4.7 Symptom expression and outcome of acute hepatitis B in adults. This figure illustrates that milder clinical disease results in a high carrier rate.

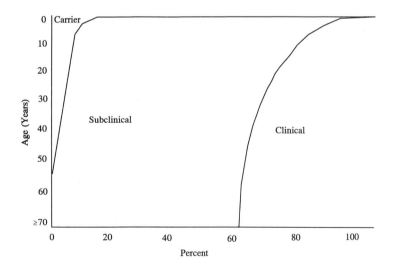

Figure 4.8 The relationahip between age and outcome after acute HBV infection. Used with permission. Hollinger FB. Hepatitis B virus. In: Hollinger FB, Robinson WS, Purcell RH, et al. eds. *Viral Hepatitis*. New York: Raven Press, 1991: 73–138.

storage for 15 years at -20°C; three to four weeks on a dried glass surface at room temperature; and for four hours at 60°C. HBV has been shown to withstand ultraviolet radiation, benzalkonium chloride and alcohol. Conversely, it is inactivated by glutaraldehyde, formalin, and urea.[14]

The HBV virus is present in all body secretions including saliva, tears, semen, vaginal secretions and breast milk. All of these secretions should be considered infectious. Only feces are considered to have negligible amounts of virus.[37]

Both percutaneous and nonpercutaneous modes of transmission occur (Figure 4.9). Percutaneous exposure (direct blood to blood contact across an interrupted barrier of skin or mucous membrane) is easier to define and understand. Examples are receiving contaminated blood products, sharing unsterilized needles, tatooing or health care accidents. Splashing of blood in the eyes or sharing toothbrushes or razors are less apparent modes of percutaneous exposure.[14, 38]

Perinatal transmission of HBV from mother to child at the time of birth is the most common mode of HBV acquisition in the world. Most chronic carriers in the Orient and Africa obtain their infection at birth. The development of HBV markers in the neonate is consistent with transmission at the time of birth when blood is known to mix between mother and child; furthermore, 95% of potential infections from mothers who have HBV can be prevented with active and passive prophylaxis at the time of birth. The vaccine and immunoglobulin would not be nearly so efficacious if HBV transmission were to occur at an earlier time in-utero.

The strongest factor to predict whether the baby will become infected is the presence or absence of the *e* antigen. Mothers who are HBeAg positive at the time of delivery will transmit the infection about 90% of the time to their untreated infants while mothers who HBsAg positive but HBeAg negative and anti-HBe positive will only transmit infection to about 10% of their untreated offspring.

Needlestick injuries from known HBsAg donors are also influenced by HBeAg status. When the donor is HBeAg positive the recipient has a 20% chance of becoming infected compared with a 1% infection rate from HBeAg negative, but HBsAg positive donors.[2]

Hepatitis B, even before blood donor screening, accounted for only 25% of post-transfusion hepatitis.[39] It is now thought to account for < 5% of cases of post-transfusion hepatitis. When HBV is transmitted through tranfusions, it is due to a low titer form of HBsAg that tests falsely negative on the EIA or RIA test. IgG or IgM anti-HBc will be the only serological marker in the patient with post-transfusion hepatitis due to HBV.

Health care workers (HCW) with acute or chronic HBV rarely transmit HBV to their patients. Risk of transmission to patients is greatest in those specialties who can accidently cut themselves such as surgeons and dentists. Even so, health care personnel with chronic HBV appear to present very little risk to their patients. A detailed review of handling the HCW infected with HBV is contained in the July 12, 1991 issue of MMWR.[40] On the other hand, more than 10,000 health care workers are estimated to become infected with HBV each year. Preventing infection in the HCW is detailed in chapter seven.

Nonpercutaneous exposure is more difficult to define. The clearest situation in which nonpercutaneous transmission occurs is during sexual activity. A high level of HBV markers exist in female prostitutes. 3% of female prostitutes in the United States are chronic carriers of HBsAg and 56% show evidence of a serologic marker for HBV. Risk is proportional to the number of lifetime sexual partners.[41]

50–95% of male homosexuals have evidence of past or present infection with HBV. Practices related to anal intercourse correlate most strongly with HBV serologic markers.[42] However, much of the infection among homosexuals may be *de facto* parenteral transmission. Rerner, et al., demonstrated multiple punctate bleeding points within the first 6 cm of the anal verge in male homosexuals; and from these bleeding points, feces, and anal canal mucosa all become contaminated with HBsAg.[43]

It is not clear that oral exposure, except in large amounts as in a laboratory pipetting accident, can transmit HBV. Oral infection apparently does not occur through the intestinal tract but through small breaks postulated to regularly exist in the oral mucosa. Attempts at experimental transmission of HBV to chimpanzees failed when the virus was placed directly into the stomach but were successful when an oral spray of infected material was applied after their gums were brushed lightly with a toothbrush.[43] In addition, pepsin and hydrochloric acid, components of gastric secretion, inactivate the virus.

The pattern of epidemics due to hepatitis B is not consistent with the fecal-oral pattern known to occur with the hepatitis A virus. For example, even though shellfish can be passively contaminated with HBV, published outbreaks of shellfish associated hepatitis have not been from type B virus.

Members of the same household are at significant risk of contracting HBV if a chronic carrier lives in the same environment.[38] Mechanisms for non-percutaneous transmission remain poorly understood.

The practical import of understanding transmission modes is to prevent infection. The use of condoms and other prevention for hepatitis B is reviewed in Chapter 5. Condoms can leak and saliva has been shown to be infectious; therefore, reliance on the use of condoms alone is not sufficient to prevent the transmission of hepatitis B. Sexual partners need to be evaluated for vaccination and hepatitis B immune globulin use.

Medical Advice for Patients with Acute Hepatitis B

Medical advice to patients with acute hepatitis B is similar to that of hepatitis A and is at the end of this chapter. One difference between HAV and HBV is that the patient with acute HBV will often be ill for a longer period of time. Patients are often ill one to two months as opposed to one to four weeks with acute HAV disease.

In addition to immunoprophylaxis of sexual contacts with HBIG, HBV vaccine is indicated for many situations detailed in Chapter 7.

Acute Hepatitis B Evaluation and Treatment Summary

1. The detection of HBsAg and anti-HBc IgM antibody are usually diagnostic of acute hepatitis B.
2. Evaluate patient for severity of disease:
    *   Prothrombin status
    *   Mental status
    *   If prothrombin time and mental status are normal, patient may be followed as outpatient. First follow-up visit within seven days.
3. Prevent secondary cases (Chapter 7).
    *   All household and sexual contacts should be evaluated for vaccine need.
    *   Sexual contacts should avoid relations until need and receipt of HBIG and vaccine occur.
    *   All body fluids are potentially infectious.
4. Make patient recommendations.
    *   Activity and bedrest as desired.
    *   Emphasize calories in AM since appetite is better.
    *   Prohibit alcohol for one year.
    *   Discontinue all meds possible until patient is well.
    *   Avoid elective surgery.
    *   Jaundice commonly lasts from one to four weeks.

Aultman Hospital
Health Sciences Library

160818

- Patients are usually off work for duration of jaundice but this recommendation varies with their type of job.
5. Report case to local health department.

References

1. Yoffe B, Noonan CA. Hepatitis B virus: new and evolving issues. *Dig Dis* 1992; 37:1–9.

2. Millman I, Eisenstein TK, Blumberg BS, eds. *Hepatitis B: the virus, the disease, and the vaccine*. New York: Plenum Press, 1984.

3. Mulley AG, Silverstein MD, Dienstag JL. Indications for use of hepatitis B vaccine, based on cost-effectiveness analysis. *N Engl J Med* 1982; 307:644–652.

4. Seeff LB, Beebe GW, Hoofnagle JH, et al. A serologic follow-up of the 1942 epidemic of post-vaccination hepatitis in the United States army. *N Engl J Med* 1987; 316:965–970.

5. Barker LF, Murray R. Acquisition of hepatitis-associated antigen. *JAMA* 1971; 216:1970–1976.

6. Hoofnagle JH, Seeff LB, Bales ZB, et al. Serologic responses in hepatitis B. In: Vyas GN, Cohen SN, Schmid R, eds. *Viral Hepatitis*. Philadelphia: Franklin Institute Press, 1978:219–242.

7. Hayman JM, Read WA. Some clinical observations on an outbreak of jaundice following yellow fever vaccination. *Am J Med Sci* 1945; 209:281–300.

8. Hollinger FB. Hepatitis B virus. In: Hollinger FB, Robinson WS, Purcell RH. *Viral Hepatitis*. New York: Raven Press, 1991:73–138.

9. Duffy J, Lidsky MD, Sharp JT, et al. Polyarthritis, polyarteritis and hepatitis B. *Medicine* 1976; 55:19–37.

10. McCarty DJ, Ormiste V. Arthritis and HB Ag-positive hepatitis. *Arch Intern Med* 1973; 132:264–268.

11. Weiss TD, Tsai CC, Baldassare AR, et al. Skin lesions in viral hepatitis. *Am J Med* 1978; 64:269–273.

12. McElguan PS. Dermatologic manifestations of hepatitis B virus infection. *J Am Acad Dermatol* 1983; 8:539–548.

13. Brooks BR. Viral hepatitis B presenting with seizure. *JAMA* 1977; 237:472–473.

14. Seeff LB. Diagnosis, therapy, and prognosis of viral hepatitis. In: Zakin D, Boyer TD, eds. *Hepatology: a textbook of liver disease*. Philadelphia. WB Saunders, 1990.

15. Koff RS, Sax DS, Freiburger Z, et al. Peripheral motor neuropathy associated with viral hepatitis. *Gastroenterology* 1973; 65:(abstract)/553.

16. Ursell PC, Habib A, Sharma P, et al. Hepatitis B virus and myocarditis. *Human Path* 1984; 15:481–484.
17. Geokas MC, Olsen H, Swanson V, et al. The association of viral hepatitis and acute pancreatitis. *West J Med* 1972; 117:1–7.
18. Achord JL. Acute pancreatitis with infectious hepatitis. *JAMA* 1968; 205:129–132.
19. Shimoda T, Shikata T, Karasawa T, et al. Light microscopic localization of hepatitis B virus antigens in the human pancreas. *Gastroenterology* 1981; 81:998–1005.
20. Alexander JA, Demetrius AJ, Gavaler JS, et al. Pancreatitis following liver transplantation. *Transplantation* 1988; 45:1062–1065.
21. Hoofnagle JH. Acute viral hepatitis: clinical features, laboratory findings, and treatment. In: Berk JE, ed. *Bockus Gastroenterology*. Philadelphia: WB Saunders, 1985: 2856–2901.
22. Wilkinson SP, Davies MH, Portmann, et al. Renal failure in otherwise uncomplicated acute viral hepatitis. *Br Med J* 1978; 2:338–341.
23. Seeff LB, Cuccherini BA, Zimmerman HJ, et al. Acetaminophen hepatoxicity in alcoholics. *Ann Intern Med* 1986; 104:399–404.
24. Kew MC, Purves LR, Bersohn I. Serum alpha-fetoprotein levels in acute viral hepatitis. *Gut* 1973; 14:939–942.
25. Karvountzis GG, Redeker AG. Relation of alpha-fetoprotein in acute hepatitis to severity and prognosis. *Ann Intern Med* 1974; 80:156–160.
26. Krugman S, Overby LR, Mushahwar IK, et al. Viral hepatitis, type B: studies on natural history and prevention reexamined. *N Engl J Med* 1979; 300:101–106.
27. Robinson WS. Biology of human hepatitis viruses. In: Zakim D, Boyer TD, eds. *Hepatology: a textbook of liver disease*. Philadelphia: WB Saunders, 1990.
28. Gitnick G. Immunoglobulin M hepatitis B core antibody: to titer or not to titer? To use or not to use? *Gastroenterology* 1983; 84:653–655.
29. Carey WD, Patel G. Viral hepatitis in the 1990's, part I: current principles of management. *Cleve Clinic J Med* 1992; 59:317–325.
30. Koff RS, Galumbos JT. Viral hepatitis. In: Schiff L, Schiff ER, eds. *Diseases of the liver*. Philadelphia: JB Lippincott, 1987.
31. Ware AJ, Eigenbrodt EH, Combes B. Prognostic significance of subacute hepatic necrosis in acute hepatitis. *Gastroenterology* 1975 ;68:519–524.
32. Seeff LB, Koff RS. Evolving concepts of the clinical and serologic consequences of hepatitis B virus infection. *Semin Liver Dis* 1986; 6:11–22.

33. Sampliner RE. The duration of hepatitis B surface antigenemia. *Arch Intern Med* 1979; 139:145–146.

34. Alward WL, McMahon BJ, Hall DB, et al. The long-term serological course of asymptomatic hepatitis B virus carriers and the development of primary hepatocellular carcinoma. *J Infect Dis* 1985; 151:604–609.

35. Redeker AG. Viral hepatitis: clinical aspects. *Am J Med Sci* 1975; 270:9–16.

36. Seeff LB, Ishak KG, Gerber MA. Unresolved clinical issues and histopathologic and immunologic aspects of chronic active hepatitis B and C. In: Lemon SM, Margolis H, eds. *Viral hepatitis and liver disease: proceedings of the 1990 International symposium on Viral Hepatitis and Liver Disease: contemporary issues and future prospects.* Baltimore: Williams and Wilkins, 1991:805–813.

37. Villarejos VM, Visona KA, Gutierrez A, et al. Role of saliva, urine and feces in the transmission of type B hepatitis. *N Eng J Med* 1974; 291:1375–1378.

38. Mitch WE, Wands JR, Maddrey WC. Hepatitis B transmission in a family. *JAMA* 1974; 227:1043–1044.

39. Seeff LB. Transfusion-associated hepatitis B: past and present. *Transfusion Med Rev* 1988; 2:204–214.

40. Centers for Disease Control. Recommendations for preventing transmission of human immunodeficiency virus and hepatitis B to patients during exposure-prone invasive procedures. *MMWR* 1991; 40: number RR-8.

41. Rosenblum L, Darrow W, Wilte J, et al. Sexual practices in the transmission of hepatitis B virus and prevalence of hepatitis delta virus infection in female prostitutes in the United States. *JAMA* 1992; 267:2477–2481.

42. Kingsley LA, Rinaldo CR, Lyter DW, et al. Sexual transmission efficiency of hepatitis B virus and human immunodeficiency virus among homosexual men. *JAMA* 1990; 264:230–234.

43. Reiner NE, Judson FN, Bond WW, et al. Asymptomatic rectal mucosal lesions and hepatitis B surface antigen at sites of sexual contact in homosexual men with persistent hepatitis B infection. *Ann Intern Med* 1984; 96:170–173.

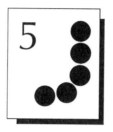

Chronic Hepatitis B

Pathology
Clinical Evaluation
Natural History
Extrahepatic Manifestations
Medical Advice

Pathology

Chronic hepatitis B is defined as persistence of the hepatitis B virus in a host for more than six months. Spontaneous resolution of HBV occurs at a very low annual rate after this period of time. A majority of carriers are asymptomatic and will not develop chronic liver disease. Hepatocellular carcinoma or extrahepatic syndromes such as polyarteritis nodosa or membranous glomerulopathy can develop regardless of symptoms referable to the liver.

Three-quarters of HBV carriers have little histological damage when biopsied. Many have normal histology or findings which suggest *chronic persistent hepatitis* (CPH). CPH is an entity where there is no significant damage to the overall architecture of the liver and mononuclear cells do not erode the limiting plate of the portal triad (Figures 5.1A & B). CPH is not associated with significant fibrosis.

To discuss pathology in chronic HBV is not to indicate that liver biopsies are mandatory. Clinically, the patient with little histological

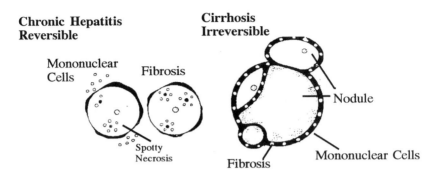

Figure 5.1A In chronic hepatitis the zonal architecture of the liver is preserved. In cirrhosis, nodular regeneration leads to loss of the hepatic architecture. Chronic hepatitis is essentially reversible, cirrhosis is not.

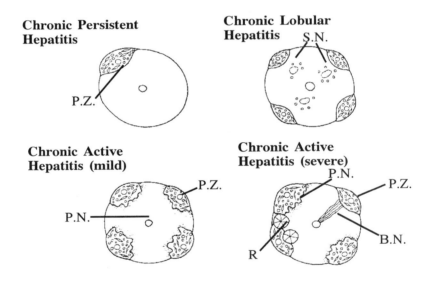

Figure 5.1B Chronic hepatitis may be divided into three types. Chronic persistent has a good prognosis. Chronic active is divided into a mild and a severe form. Chronic lobular hepatitis P.Z. = portal zone; S.N. = spotty necrosis; P.N. = piecemeal necrosis; B.N.= bridging necrosis. R = rosettes. Figures 5.1 A & B used with permission. Sherlock S. Diseases of the Liver and Biliary System. Oxford. Blackwell Scientific.1989. p 340.

damage will have minimal elevation of aminotransferase levels, a normal serum albumin level and lack physical findings of chronic liver disease. This clinical picture is referred to as the *healthy* carrier state emphasizing that these patients are asymptomatic and probably not at risk of progressive liver disease. However, controversy exists about using the word *healthy* to describe these patients since they may still develop hepatocellular carcinoma and transmit the virus. Nonetheless, this writer favors the term when talking to patients since it reduces anxiety about their disease and prognosis.

The second pathological and clinical outcome of the chronic HBV status which occurs in about one quarter of carriers is one of progressive liver disease. Histologically, this can be manifested by significant fibrosis and erosion of the portal triad limiting plate by mononuclear cells in a picture referred to as *piecemeal necrosis*(Figure 5.1). Overall, these findings are referred to as *chronic active hepatitis*(CAH). Cirrhosis may develop in as many as 50% of adult patients with CAH. While cirrhosis can develop within the first year, the estimated annual incidence in adults with CAH is 2.4% (China)[1] to 5.9% (Italy)[2]. Cirrhosis seldom occurs in children with chronic active hepatitis (Chapter 6). The five year survival in the United States for CPH, CAH, and CAH with cirrhosis is 97%, 86% and 55%, respectively (Figure 5.2).[3] In a follow-up

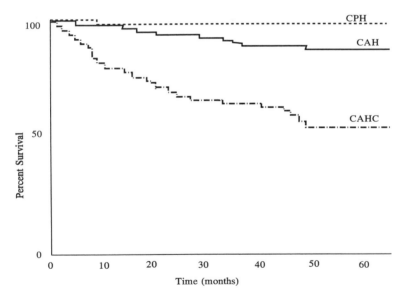

Figure 5.2 Survival of chronic hepatitis B Kaplan-Meier 5-year survival curves for 379 patients with chronic hepatitis B. The dash-dot line gives the duration of survival for 130 patients with chronic active hepatitis and cirrhosis (CAHC); the solid line represents the survival curve for 128 patients with chronic active hepatitis (CAH); the dash line gives the survival data for 121 patients with chronic persistent hepatitis (CPH). Each of these curves is significantly different from the others at p < 0.001.[2] (Reproduced with permission, from Weissberg JI, et al. Survival in chronic hepatitis B· *Ann Intern Med* 1984; 101:613–616.

to the latter study, the fifteen year survival for these groups are estimated to be 77%, 66% and 40%.[4] The patient with progressive liver disease but not yet cirrhosis often has few symptoms; fatigue may be the only symptom present.

»   *The current histological system has been used since an international group of liver experts established nomenclature in 1968.[5] The following section includes comments about terminology which may not interest the general reader. It is included to help readers understand current reports in this area.*

Two objections, lack of etiology and variable prognosis have troubled current thinkers.[5, 6] Some wish to replace the terms *chronic persistent hepatitis* and *chronic active hepatitis* with mild chronic hepatitis due to hepatitis B (or other cause)" and "severe chronic hepatitis due to hepatitis B".[6] Ludwig has proposed a four point system for inflammatory activity and a separate four point system for fibrosis along with etiology (Figure 5.1). In addition, Ludwig has called for an international nomenclature group. The problem with such a change is that the complexity of such a system would turn the understanding of viral hepatitis into a province only for specialists. The intricacy of lymphoma classification looms as a warning to those wishing to change nomenclature. Certainly, adding etiology to a morphological description is an improvement. This means, as it should, the clinician and pathologist need to work together.

Pathologists have worried about whether morphology predicts prognosis. Certainly, "chronic active hepatitis" has a different prognosis depending on whether hepatitis B (worse) or hepatitis C (better) is present. While the presence of "piecemeal necrosis" is an important determination of classification, the *sine qua non* of progressive liver disease is the presence of fibrosis on biopsy.[7] Ludwig reminds us that an integral part of the original concept behind "persistent" vs "active" designation was the clinical picture.[5] Unfortunately, these terms have evolved into a morphological diagnosis only.

Adding an etiology to a histological diagnosis seems reasonable. The author hopes that future classification systems are not too complex. The current work will retain the classic designations of "chronic persistent" versus "chronic active" hepatitis since all of the viral hepatitis literature until now has used these terms.

Table 5.1 Proposal for an updated terminology of chronic viral hepatitis. Used with permission. Ludwig J. The nomenclature of chronic active hepatitis: an obituary. *Gastroenterology* 1993; 105:276. Table modified.

Etiological Designations	Grade of Inflammatory Activity			Stage/Degree of Fibrosis	
Chronic hepatitis	*Grade*	*Portal*	*Lobular*	*Stage*	*Degree of Fibrosis*
Chronic hepatitis B	0	None / minimal	None	1	No fibrosis or fibrosis confined to enlarged portal tracts
Chronic hepatitis B & D					
Chronic hepatitis C					
Chronic viral hepatitis, type unspecified	1	Portal inflammation (CPH)	Inflammation but no necrosis	2	Periportal fibrosis or portal-to-portal septa but intact architecture
	2	Mild limiting plate necrosis (mild CAH)	Focal necrosis or acidophilic bodies	3	Septal fibrosis with architectural distortion, no obvious cirrhosis
	3	Moderate limiting plate necrosis (moderate CAH)	Severe focal cell damage		
	4	Severe limiting plate necrosis (severe CAH)	Damage includes bridging necrosis	4	Probable or definite cirrhosis

Clinical Evaluation

The clinicians role in evaluating patients with chronic hepatitis B is to distinguish between those patients with mild disease or a "healthy" carrier state from those with progressive liver disease. Alfa- interferon therapy is available for selected patients with progressive liver disease.

To properly classify patients, the evaluator needs to inquire about fatigue and ability to work. The physical examination should look for stigmata of chronic liver disease such as spider angiomata, splenomegaly or hepatomegaly. Laboratory clues which suggest a progressive chronic liver disease include low serum albumin, aminotransferases greater than 200 IU/L and a platelet count of < 140,000.[8, 11] A positive HBeAg correlates with a high viral replication and a more severe histological picture. Conversely, if the anti-Hbe marker is present, the patient will have little or no viral replication and will often have a mild to normal histological picture.

Many patients are simple to classify on a clinical basis with the foregoing approach. Occasionally, a patient with mixed findings will present. In the grey area, between those who have mild disease and those who have severe disease, a liver biopsy can be helpful. At a recent conference of hepatologists interested in viral hepatitis, a wide variety of opinion was expressed as to what the indications for liver biopsy are in hepatitis B, if any. The most useful question about performing a biopsy in hepatitis B is: Will it change what we are going to do? If the answer is yes, then it is reasonable to perform it.

Natural History of Chronic Hepatitis B

The designation of *chronic carrier* should not imply a permanent state. The natural history of chronic HBV is one of slow but step-wise clearance in many patients.

The chronic carrier is first positive for HBsAg and HBeAg with high levels of HBV DNA indicating intensive viral replication. Significant liver damage may or may not occur during this phase. The active replication phase may last one to twenty years or longer (Figure 5.3)

The second step in clearing the virus involves seroconversion of HBeAg to its antibody, anti-Hbe. An acute exacerbation of clinical hepatitis can happen at the time of *e* antigen loss; an exacerbation that can mimic a de novo attack of acute hepatitis B with the exception that the anti-Hbe marker is present. The annual rate of HBeAg converting to anti-HBs has been reported to range from 2.7% to 25%.[10] Coincident with seroconversion, HBV DNA levels decline and aminotransferase levels fall or normalize. The HBV virus replicates at low levels during the HBsAg positive, anti-Hbe positive phase. Low levels of replication predict diminished infectivity and mild liver injury. The liver becomes less inflamed, and if cirrhosis has not occurred during the prior active replication phase, it will not develop during the low viral replication stage.

The HBeAg negative, HBsAg positive and anti-Hbe phase is not always stable. *Reactivation* of the *e* antigen can occur with a clinical picture that will also mimic acute viral hepatitis(Figure 5.3). Chemotherapeutic agents for malignant or non-malignant disease have reactivated the *e* antigen, sometimes with fatal results.[10, 11] Immunosuppression associated with organ transplantation has been associated with reactivation. Withdrawal of short courses of corticosteroids,

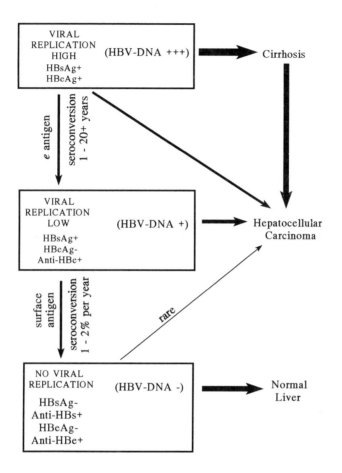

Figure 5.3 Natural history of chronic hepatitis B.

even outside the transplantation setting, has also caused reactivation.[10] Cellular studies show that HBV DNA contains a glucocorticoid-responsive element that helps to mediate expression of HBV genes in infected mammalian cells.[12]

More troublesome is that reactivation can take place spontaneously. In one report, 8 of 25 HBsAg positive, anti-Hbe positive patients over a 14 month period developed the abrupt onset of symptoms, aminotransferase elevations and the reappearance of *e* antigen. One of the eight patients died.[13]

Non-Progressive HBV Disease

Mild hepatitis, CPH, CAH
and
HBeAg$^-$ or HBV-DNA$^-$

Progress to Cirrhosis Uncertain

CAH > CPH
and
HBeAg$^+$ or HBV-DNA$^+$

- Improved histology with loss of
  e antigen can also occur

- Older (> age 40) patients are more
  likely to progress

Progress to Cirrhosis Predictable

Severe CAH (bridging necrosis) with HBeAg$^+$ or HBV-DNA$^+$

Figure 5.4 Natural history of chronic hepatitis B in adults. CPH = chronic persistent hepatitis. CAH = chronic active hepatitis.

Unless one knows that a patient has previously been a carrier for HBV, it is difficult to distinguish e antigen seroconversion or reactivation from a *de novo* attack of acute hepatitis B. It is helpful if the anti-HBc IgM antibody is negative but instances of this antibody occasionally being present in either seroconversion or reactivation are reported.[14]

The final stage of the carrier state is disappearance of surface antigen. HBsAg converts to anti-HBs at the rate of 1–2% per year.[10] Biochemical tests normalize and histology becomes normal unless irreversible damage occurred earlier. The patient is considered non-infectious when anti-HBs appears.

A more specific natural history for an individual patients can be predicted from a combination of *viral status* and *host response*.

Viral status refers to the degree of viral replication. Until recently, the "e" antigen-antibody system was utilized to describe the amount of hepatitis B viral replication; e antigen positive patients have significant viral replication and e antigen negative/e antibody positive patients usually have little or no active HBV replication. However, introduction of a new assay of HBV replication by molecular hybridization, called HBV-DNA, helps to delineate HBV status more directly. A total of six studies have shown HBV-DNA to be present in 83 to 100% of HBV carriers with e antigen (HBeAg+) and in 26 to 64% of e antigen negative/e antibody positive (HBeAg⁻/anti-Hbe⁺) patients.[15] Thus, while the presence of e antigen has a high correlation with ongoing viral replication, the absence of e antigen and the presence of e antibody has poor correlation with complete disappearance of HBV replication.

Host response refers to the histological picture discussed earlier in the chapter. Advancing pathological stages are often, but not invariably, associated with a poorer prognosis. Combining the e antigen status (or HBV-DNA status) and the pathological picture allows a more precise prognosis than using either parameter alone. The natural history of three groups of patients has now been delineated: one, asymptomatic patients with persistently normal ALT and HBeAg⁻; two, non-cirrhotic patients with chronic hepatitis and elevated ALT values; and, three, patients with cirrhosis.

A ten year follow-up study of 92 asymptomatic Italian HBV carriers discovered by blood donor screening has been done.[16] Subjects were principally HBeAg⁻ (88 negative, 4 positive) and had persistently normal ALT values at baseline and in 85% of patients on follow-up. Ten of 60 subjects tested were positive for HBV-DNA. During a mean follow-up of 130 months, only one of 91 patients developed cirrhosis and no liver-related deaths occurred. The one patient in whom cirrhosis developed was thought to be caused by alcohol use.[16]

In patients with chronic hepatitis, Fattovich et al.[17] followed 44 patients with *chronic persistent hepatitis* (CPH), a pathological stage felt to have a better prognosis than *chronic active hepatitis* (CAH). 38 subjects were HBV-DNA positive (31 HBeAg⁺, 7 anti-Hbe⁺). 12 (32%) of these 38 patients progressed to CAH (six cases) or active cirrhosis (six cases) during a mean histologic follow-up of 4.2 years. 21 in this group were unchanged and five cases improved to a normal histologic appearance. None of the six anti-Hbc positive/HBV-DNA negative group progressed on follow-up biopsy and one subject improved to normal.

Another study by Fattovich et al. showed that the presence of severe CAH, as manifested by bridging hepatic necrosis, and continuing viral replication were the most important risk factors for the development of cirrhosis.[2]

The age of the patient with chronic HBV is also very important in determining progression. Pediatric patients are much more likely to lose viral replication and not progress to cirrhosis as compared to adult patients. The natural history of HBV infection in children is discussed in Chapter 6. In adult patients, age over 40 has been associated with a greater likelihood of progressive disease.[2, 18]

Cirrhosis due to HBV can have markedly different survival depending on a number of factors. In order of frequency, the causes of death for these patients are: hepatocellular carcinoma, liver failure and upper gastrointestinal bleeding. The strongest pessimistic prognostic factors are: age, elevated bilirubin levels and presence of ascites.[18] Marked declines in survival occur in patients at ages 36, 50 and 60. A bilirubin even mildly elevated at 1–2 mg/dl (13–34 µmol/L) predicts poorer survival. Decompensated cirrhosis is defined as the presence of ascites, encephalopathy, bilirubin level ≥ 2 mg/dl (> 34 µmol/L), or a history of variceal bleeding. Patients with decompensated cirrhosis have a five year survival of 14% versus 84% with compensated cirrhosis.[18]

HBeAg predicts survival in patients with compensated cirrhosis. e antigen positive patients have a 72% five year survival versus 97% in e antigen negative patients. For patients who seroconvert the e antigen during observation, there is a 2.2-fold decrease in the death rate.[18]

Cirrhosis appears ten years earlier in HBV carriers who are daily users of alcohol. A ten year follow-up study shows that carriers who are habitual users of alcohol have a significantly shorter lifespan than abstainers.[19] Even small amounts of daily alcohol use cause significantly higher aminotransferase levels in chronic HBsAg carriers as compared to controls (Figure 5.5).[20]

Extrahepatic Manifestations

Polyarteritis nodosa and glomerulonephritis are uncommon extrahepatic manifestations of chronic hepatitis B.

Polyarteritis nodosa

Polyarteritis nodosa (PAN) is a systemic arteritis involving small and medium arteries. Numerous manifestations can occur such as arthralgias, fever, abdominal pain, renal disease, central nervous system abnormalities or mononeuritis multiplex. The frequency of clinically recognized PAN is very low. In a hemodialysis unit, it occurred in 3 of 266 HBsAg positive patients, and in a needle induced HBV epidemic, 1 of 301 patients developed PAN.[21]

A majority of patients with established PAN are HBsAg positive. If sensitive assays such as monoclonal antibodies or HBV DNA levels are

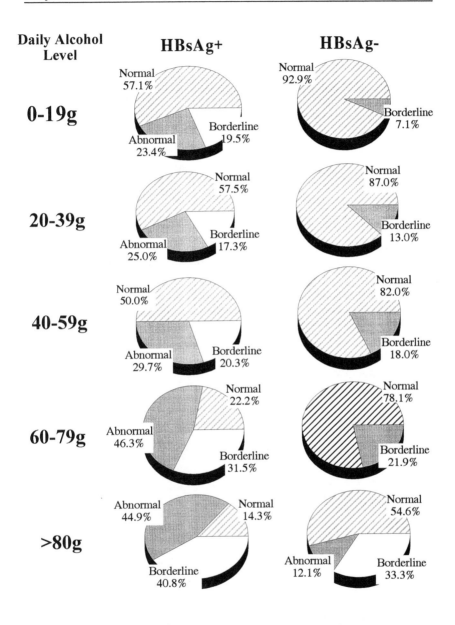

Figure 5.5 Prevalence of liver abnormalities according to daily ethanol intake. *Borderline values* are elevated aminotransferase values not exceeding twice normal and/or hepatomegaly of not more than 14 cm; findings beyond these limits are *abnormal*. Results are statistically different at every ethanol level use between HBsAg carriers and controls. Used with permission. Villa E, et al. Susceptibility of chronic symptomless HBsAg carriers to ethanol induced hepatic damage. Volume 2: 1243-4, ©*The Lancet Ltd.*, 1982.

used, as many as 79% of unselected PAN patients have evidence for chronic hepatitis B infection.[22]

The pathogenesis of PAN consists of immune complexes of surface antigen and surface antibody depositing in arterioles and arteries.[23] Angiography is diagnostic if microaneurysms are seen in arterioles of multiple organs such as kidney or liver.

The mortality rate is 40% in three years whether or not the patient is HBsAg positive.[24] If the patient survives the initial severity of illness, the long-term prognosis appears good. Boyer, et al, report a five year follow-up on three patients who became clinically well despite continued carriage of HBsAg.[25] The hepatitis B surface antigen in patients with PAN seems to rarely, if ever, disappear.[21]

Corticosteroid or cytotoxic agents have been suggested for treatment of HBV-PAN in uncontrolled trials. However, many of these patients developed severe hepatitis while on these medications suggesting that the corticosteroid or cytotoxic therapy increased viral replication.[26]

Alfa-interferon treatment of patients with PAN is not yet reported. Concern over acceleration of immune complex injury with alfa-interferon treatment has been raised.[21] Plasmapheresis and adenosine arabinoside are reported to be beneficial in HBV-PAN.[26, 27]

Glomerulonephritis

Glomerulopathy takes a number of forms in hepatitis B. The most common clinical finding is the nephrotic syndrome with the most prevalent pathological finding on kidney biopsy being membranous glomerulopathy (HBVMN).

All three HBV antigens, HBsAg, HBeAg and HBcAg, have been localized by immunofluorescence in the glomerular capillary wall of patients with HBVMN. This would support a mechanism whereby immune complexes containing HBV are localized in the subepithelial space either as a result of passive trapping or local formation of immune complex.[29]

HBVMN is considered to be a rare complication of hepatitis B. McMahon's prospective study of 7815 carrier-years in an Alaskan population found one case of glomerulopathy.[30] However, in series of patients who are reported with glomerulonephritis, the prevalence of HBV infection ranges from 11 to 56%. The prevalence of HBV varies as to whether HBV is endemic to the country reporting the series.[24]

The natural history of HBVMN is different for children and adults. Spontaneous remission may occur in 30–60% of children though they can remain symptomatic for up to 12 months.[31] Spontaneous remission in adults does not occur but proteinuria tends to decrease over time.[31]

Corticosteroids are contraindicated since viral replication increases during their use.[28, 31, 32]

Biochemical and serological remission has been reported in four adult patients with HBVMN treated with alfa interferon for four months.[33] Importantly, three of these four patients had acquired HBV in their adult life through sexual or intravenous transmission. In five patients from Hong Kong with HBV infection since childhood, only one patient treated with alpha interferon had a complete remission with seroconversion of HBeAg to anti-Hbe.[33] The National Institutes of Health has reported treating fourteen patients with HBV related glomerulopathy. Alpha-interferon treatment for 16 weeks caused loss of HBeAg and HBV-DNA from serum in 64% of patients with marked, progressive improvement in the nephrotic syndrome in those who responded.[34] Alpha interferon treatment of pediatric patients with HBVMN has not been reported.

Hepatocellular carcinoma

Chronic HBV infection can lead to the development of hepatocellular carcinoma (HCC). The geographical distribution of HCC correlates with the prevalence of HBV infection. Since the prevalence of infection of HBV is highest in Southeast Asia and sub-Saharan Africa, hepatocellular carcinoma is the most common cancer in males throughout the world.[35] It is estimated that more than 500,000 deaths occur annually due to HCC.[36]

The largest prospective study of the development of HCC in HBV carriers was undertaken in Taiwan. 22,707 middle aged males were tested for HBsAg carrier status and were followed for one to five years for the development of HCC. Of the 3,454 positive for HBsAg, 113 men (3.2%) developed HCC compared to three of 19,253 HBsAg negative men. The relative risk in HBV carriers was estimated to be 223 times that of non-carriers.[37] Other prospective studies have reported relative risks ranging from 15 to 307.[38]

A relative risk of > 200 needs to be placed in perspective. For example, if a patient smokes two packs of cigarettes per day for 50 years, the relative risk of developing lung cancer is only ten-fold. Thus, the risk of HCC in HBV disease is 20x the risk of lung cancer developing in heavy smokers. However, development of HCC is not inevitable in chronic carriers. The life-time risk of HCC is probably much less than 10%.

HCC patients with HBV typically have low titers of HBsAg and are HBeAg negative/anti-HBe positive indicating low levels of viremia and long duration of infection. Age distribution of HCC patients suggests that these tumors appear after a mean duration of 35 years. HCC is rare in children.[37] Most cases of HCC occur above age 55 in the United States and Europe.

Tumor development (i.e. oncogenesis) occurs as a result of HBV DNA integration into the host's hepatocyte genome.[39] Integrations have been found on human chromosomes 6, 9, 11, 17 and 18.[15]

Cirrhosis, alcohol ingestion and cigarette smoking are co-factors for the development of HCC. Most patients with HCC due to HBV have co-existing cirrhosis. Studies have shown that HCC coexists with cirrhosis 60–86% of the time.[40] The average age of patients with HCC who drink alcohol regularly is 48.9 years versus 61.4 years in non-drinkers.[41]

The habitual alcohol user is felt to have 3.4× the risk of HCC compared to abstainers. A dose-response relationship between cigarette smoking and HCC occurs with an odds ratio of 1.1, 1.5 and 2.6, respectively, for those who smoke 1–10, 11–20 and more than 20 cigarettes a day.[42]

In addition to HCC, chronic HBV infection may predispose to other cancers. Olatuji et al.[43] report a 36% prevalence of HBsAg in malignant lymphoproliferative disorders compared to 8% in their control population.

Detailed treatment of HCC is beyond the scope of this book. Briefly, the cancer is usually advanced at the time of diagnosis with an average time of survival of four months. Radiation therapy is not indicated since normal hepatocytes are more sensitive to radiation than are tumor cells. Systemic chemotherapy has a low response rate and high side effect profile. New approaches with angiographic embolization of chemotherapy agents appear to improve survival to one year in some patients. Surgical resection of limited disease is the only approach which can produce a long-term cure.[39] Few patients at the time of diagnosis have limited disease or a non-cirrhotic liver to allow an extensive resection for a cure.

For the foregoing reasons, it has been thought that asymptomatic screening of HBsAg positive carriers might find patients amenable to surgery. Screening has been advocated with either ultrasound or alpha-fetoprotein serum assays or both.

Several Oriental studies have shown that HCC can be detected before the onset of symptoms; whether earlier detection translates into increased survival remains unclear.[40] Asymptomatic screening studies must take into account lead-time bias which accounts for increased survival merely because the tumor was detected earlier.

The only Western screening study, by Columbo et al.[44] followed 417 patients with cirrhosis over five years. 355 patients had either hepatitis B or C present. Patients with normal AFP levels and ultrasound examinations at enrollment were screened yearly with these tests. Patients with mild elevation of AFP (> 20 µg/L) and normal ultrasound at enrollment were screened every three months. 29 cases of HCC were discovered but outcome did not differ between those patients who underwent surgery and those who refused surgery. Columbo concludes that their screening program did not increase the rate of potentially curable tumors.

Unfortunately, cirrhosis is usually present when HCC is discovered in an asymptomatic patient. Resection of the cirrhotic liver commonly leads to post-operative liver failure and subsequent mortality. In this author's opinion, there are no simple or reliable methods currently available for predicting post-operative survival of patients with HCC and cirrhosis.

Liver transplantation for HCC due to hepatitis B virus has a very poor survival[45] and is still considered experimental.

Screening for HCC is expensive. An ultrasound and alpha-fetoprotein test every six months costs about $500 per year for every patient. Given the uncertain benefit, high cost, and difficult to apply surgical approach, screening for HCC at the current time is unproven and unwarranted.[15, 37] In a cost sensitive environment, the effort and expense should be directed towards universal vaccination with the hepatitis B vaccine to prevent *both* HBV infection and HCC.

Medical Advice for Chronic Carriers of Hepatitis B

Chronic carriers of HBV should be checked for presence of the *e* antigen and delta antibody. The status of the HBeAg or its antibody helps to place the patient in the natural history of the disease and reveals infectivity. In addition, current eligibility for alpha interferon treatment (Chapter 8) requires the presence of the *e* antigen. Delta hepatitis can superinfect chronic carriers of HBV and is diagnosed with either an IgG or IgM antibody to delta virus (Chapter 13).

A common omission seen in referred patients to the author is the failure of evaluating members of the same household for hepatitis B vaccine eligibility (Chapter 7). If the patient has evidence of chronic liver disease, influenza vaccine is recommended yearly and the pneumococcal vaccine is given once.[46]

Alcohol should be avoided entirely and the patient's chart labelled about the hazards of receiving corticosteroids or chemotherapy agents. Other physicians caring for the patient need to be aware that these agents can fatally reactivate HBV. Corticosteroids or chemotherapeutic agents are not contraindicated but should be used judiciously. In contrast to other causes of cirrhosis, colchicine, when used in an attempt to reduce the formation of fibrosis, does not appear to improve laboratory parameters or lower mortality in hepatitis B when tested in a five year double blind trial.[47]

Finally, the patient with chronic hepatitis B should be evaluated for possible treatment with alpha-interferon (Chapter 8).

Treatment Summary—Chronic Carriers of Hepatitis B

1. Define where the patient is in the natural history of chronic HBV disease, stage the amount of current damage and determine the potential for progression to cirrhosis.
   - HBeAg, anti-Hbe status (or HBV-DNA status) is helpful.
   - If serum albumin normal, ALT near normal and patient is asymptomatic, no liver biopsy is needed. Otherwise, histology, age and viral replication status help to predict prognosis and response to alfa-interferon treatment (Chapter 8).
   - Initial visit should include ultrasound of liver to exclude hepatocellular carcinoma (HCC). Routine screening for HCC is not recommended.
   - Exclude superinfection with hepatitis C or D serology.
2. Evaluate and vaccinate, if indicated, members of the household in which the carrier resides (Chapter 7).
3. Chronic HBV carriers should:
   - Abstain from alcohol and cigarette smoking entirely.
   - Avoid corticosteroids or chemotherapeutic agents (can reactivate severe hepatitis). Chronic HBV is a relative contraindication to receiving these agents and not absolute. Label the medical chart about this risk.
   - Receive the influenza vaccine yearly and pneumococcal vaccine once, if they have evidence of chronic liver disease.

References

1. Liaw Y, Tai D, Chu C, et al. The development of cirrhosis in patients with chronic type B hepatitis: a prospective study. *Hepatology* 1988; 8:493–496.

2. Fattovich G, Brollo L, Giustina G, et al. Natural history and prognostic factors for chronic hepatitis B. *Gut* 1991; 32:294–298.

3. Weissberg JI, Andres LL, Smith CI, et al. Survival in chronic hepatitis B. *Ann Intern Med* 1984; 101:613–616.

4. Ladenheim J, Yao F, Martin MC, et al. Survival in chronic hepatitis B: a 15-year follow-up. *Hepatology* 1993; 18:199 (abstract).

5. Ludwig J. The nomenclature of chronic active hepatitis: an obituary. *Gastroenterology* 1993; 105:274–278.

6. Zetterman RK. Chronic hepatitis: is it persistent, active or just chronic? *Am J Gastroenterology* 1993; 88:1–2.

7. Lewis FW, Ready JB, Zetterman RW, et al. Methods of evaluation of the severity and prognosis of chronic liver disease. In: Rector WG, Jr, ed. *Complications of Chronic Liver Disease*. St. Louis: Mosby, 1992: 1–23.

8. Williams AL, Hoofnagle JH. Ratio of serum aspartate to alanine aminotransferase in chronic hepatitis: relationship to cirrhosis. *Gastroenterology* 1988; 95:734–739.

9. Tine F, Caltagirone M, Canama C, et al. Clinical indicants of compensated cirrhosis: a prospective study. In: Diazani MU, Gentilini P. *Chronic Liver Damage*. New York: Elsevier-Science, 1990: 187–198.

10. Seeff LB, Koff RS. Evolving concepts of the clnical and serologic consequences of hepatitis B virus infection. *Semin Liver Dis* 1986; 6:11–22.

11. Flowers MA, Heathcote J, Wanless IR, et al. Fulminant hepatitis as a consequence of reactivation of hepatitis B virus infection after discontinuation of low-dose methotrexate therapy. *Ann Intern Med* 1990; 112:381–2.

12. Tur-Kaspa R, Burk RD, Shaul Y, et al. Hepatitis B virus DNA contains a glucocorticoid-responsive element. *Proc Natl Acad Sci* 1986; 83:1627–1631.

13. Davis GL, Hoofnagle JH, Waggoner JG. Spontaneous reactivation of chronic hepatitis B virus infection. *Gastroenterology* 1984; 86:230–235.

14. Davis GL, Hoofnagle JH. Reactivation of chronic type B hepatitis presenting as acute viral hepatitis. *Ann Intern Med* 1985; 102:762–765.

15. Shafritz DA, Sherman M, Tur-kaspa R. Hepatitis B virus persistence, chronic liver disease and primary liver cancer. In: Zakim D, Boyer TD, eds. *Hepatology: a textbook of liver disease*. Philadelphia: WB Saunders, 1990: 945–957.

16. De Franchis R, Meucci G, Vecchi M, et al. The natural history of asymptomatic hepatitis B surface antigen carriers. *Ann Intern Med* 1993; 118:191–194.

17. Fattovich G, Brollo L, Alberti A, et al. Chronic persistent hepatitis B can be a progressive disease when associated with sustained virus replication. *J Hepatology* 1990; 11:29–33.

18. De Jongh F, Janssen H, DeMan R, et al. Survival and prognostic indicators in hepatitis B surface antigen-positive cirrhosis of the liver. *Gastroenterology* 1992; 103:1630–1635.

19. Shioma S, Kuroki T, Minamitani S, et al. Effect of drinking on the outcome of cirrhosis in patients with hepatitis B or C. *J Gastroenterology Hepat* 1992; 3:274–276.

20. Villa E, Barchi T, Grisendi A, et al. Susceptibility of chronic symptomless HBsAg carriers to ethanol induced hepatic damage. *Lancet* 1982; 2:1243–1244.

21. Christian CL. Hepatitis B virus and systemic vasculitis. *Clin Exp Rheum* 1991; 9:1–2.

22. Marcellin P, Calmus Y, Takahashi H, et al. Latent hepatitis B virus infection in systemic necrotizing vasculities. *Clin Exp Rheumatol* 1991; 9:23–28.

23. Michalak T. Immune complexes of hepatitis B surface antigen in the pathogenesis of periarteritis nodosa. *Am J Path* 1978; 90:619–627.

24. Seeff LB. Diagnosis, therapy and prognosis of viral hepatitis. In: Zakin D, Boyer TD, eds. *Hepatology: a textbook of liver disease.* Philadelphia: WB Saunders, 1990.

25. Boyer TD, Tong MJ, Rakela J, et al. Immunologic studies and clinical follow-up HBsAg-positive polyarteritis nodosa. *Dig Dis* 1977; 22:497–501.

26. Guillevin L. Treatment of polyarteritis nodosa and Churg-Strauss angiitis. *Prog Clin Bio Res* 1990; 309–317.

27. Trepo C, Ouzan D. Successful therapy of polyarteritis due to hepatitis B virus by combination of plasma exchanges and adenine arabinoside therapy. *Hepatology* 1985; 5:1022 (abstract)

28. Lai KN, Lai FM. Clinical features and the natural course of hepatitis B virus-related glomerulopathy in adults. *Kidney International* 1991; 40 (Suppl 35):S40–45.

29. Johnson RJ, Couser WG. Hepatitis B infection and renal disease: clinical, imunopathogenetic and therapeutic consideration. *Kidney International* 1990; 37:663–676.

30. McMahon BJ, Alberts SR, Wainwright RB, et al. Hepatitis-B related sequelae. *Arch Intern Med* 1990; 1051–1054.

31. Lin CY. Clinical features and natural course of HBV-related glomerulopathy in children. *Kidney International* 1991; 40 (Suppl 35): S46–53.

32. Lai KN, Li PK, Lui SF, et al. Membranous nephropathy related to hepatitis B virus in adults. *N Engl J Med* 1991; 324:1457–1463.

33. Lisker-Melman M, Webb D, Di Bisceglie AM, et al. Glomerulonephritis caused by hepatitis B virus infection: treatment with recombinant human alpha-interferon. *Ann Intern Med* 1989; 111:47–-83.

34. Conjeevaram H, Balow JE, Austin H, et al. Long-term follow-up of hepatitis B virus related glomerulonephritis treated with alpha interferon. *Hepatology* 1993; 18:146 (abstract).

35. Vyas GN, Blum HE. Hepatitis B virus infection: current concepts of chronicity and immunity. *West J Med* 1984; 140:754–762.

36. Hollinger FB. Hepatitis B virus. In: Hollinger FB, Robinson WS, Purcell RH. *Viral Hepatitis*. New York: Raven Press, 1991:73–138.

37. Beasley R, Lin C, Hwang L, et al. Hepatocellular carcinoma and hepatitis B virus. *Lancet* 1981; 2:1129–1132.

38. Alward WL, McMahon BJ, Hall DB, et al. The long term serological course of asymptomatic hepatitis B virus carriers and the development of primary hepatocellular carcinoma. *J Infect Dis* 1985; 151:604–609.

39. Di Bisceglie AM, Rusti VK, Hoofnagle JH, et al. Hepatocellular carcinoma: NIH Conference. *Ann Intern Med* 1988; 108:390–401.

40. Oka H, Kurioka N, Kim K, et al. Prospective study of early detection of hepatocellular carcinoma in patients with cirrhosis. *Hepatology* 1990; 12:680–87.

41. Ohnishi K, Shinji I, Iwama S, et al. The effect of chronic habitual alcohol intake on the development of liver cirrhosis and hepatocellular carcinoma. *Cancer* 1982; 49:672–77.

42. Chen C, Liang K, Chang A, et al. Effects of hepatitis B virus, alcohol drinking, cigarette smoking and familial tendency on hepatocellular carcinoma. *Hepatology* 1991; 13:398–406.

43. Olatunji P, Okpala I, Sorunmu M. Hepatitis B surface antigenaemia in patients with malignant lymphoproliferative disorders. Tokai *J Exp Clin Med* 1991; 16:171.

44. Columbo M, De Franchis R, Ninno E, et al. Hepatocellular carcinoma in Italian patients with cirrhosis. *N Engl J Med* 1991; 325:675–680.

45. Starzl TE, Demetris AJ, Van Thiel D. Liver transplantation. *N Engl J Med* 1989; 321:1092–1099.

46. Gardner P, Schaffner W. Immunization of adults. *N Eng J Med* 1993; 328:1252–1258.

47. Wang YJ, Lee SD, Tsai YT, et al. A controlled trail of colchicine in patients with hepatitis B virus related post-necrotic cirrhosis. *Hepatology* 1992; 16:68 (abstract).
48. Sherlock S. *Diseases of the Liver and Biliary System.* Oxford: Blackwell Scientific Publications, 1989:340.

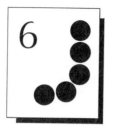

Special Circumstances with HBV

Pregnancy
Pediatrics
Difficult Serology
HIV Disease

Pregnancy

As in any kind of viral hepatitis except type E, the well nourished pregnant woman with *acute* hepatitis B fares no differently than her non-pregnant counterpart. Given the marked change in immunology that occurs during pregnancy, it is surprising that only two cases of reactivation of HBV have been reported during pregnancy.[1]

Limited data exists to suggest that pregnancy may help to clear HBV virus. Among thirteen women who were HBsAg positive and HBeAg negative during pregnancy, seven (54%) became HBsAg negative following delivery.[2] Larger samples will be needed to see if the post-partum condition helps to clear the HBV virus.

The results of pregnancy for the woman with chronic hepatitis B will depend on whether she is a "healthy" carrier or has progressive liver disease or cirrhosis. Again, the *healthy* chronic carrier will not have any unusual problems with her pregnancy compared to uninfected mothers. Congenital malformations, stillbirths, spontaneous abortions or low birth weight infants are not increased in this group. An increased risk of prematurity, however, may exist.[3]

Since the liver is a principle site of sex steroid metabolism, women with significant chronic liver disease have markedly decreased fertility; thus, few cases of pregnancy in women with cirrhosis are reported. Fetal morbidity and mortality are increased in gestations from women who have cirrhosis. The mother may experience complications of her liver disease such as bleeding esophageal varices or ascites during pregnancy. The tendency to have these complications is due to both the gravid uterus and the increased blood volume of pregnancy which work together to increase portal hypertension.[4]

The most important issue in the subject of hepatitis B and pregnancy is the prevention of post-partum infection of the neonate with HBIG and the hepatitis B vaccine. The parameters of post-natal prevention are presented in chapter seven.

Finally, the mother with peripartum acute infection or chronic HBV will have infected breast milk.[5] Beasley et al. followed 147 babies born to mothers with HBV and found no increased incidence of HBV infection in those who were breast fed.[6] However, mothers who are HBV carriers should not donate to human milk banks.

Pediatric Issues

Earlier in the book, several chapters discuss the different course hepatitis B virus takes in younger patients. To summarize these differences, the younger the patient is when HBV infection is contracted, the more likely a chronic carrier state will ensue. In addition, the lower the age at the time of acquisition of HBV, the less likely a patient will have any symptoms as a result of infection; that is, younger patients have a much greater likelihood of asymptomatic infection (Figure 6.1). Children who are chronic carriers and with or without chronic active hepatitis have normal growth patterns.[7]

Horizontal transmission (i.e. between same-aged peers) is common in children. Children born in the U. S. to Southeast Asian refugees have a tenfold rate of HBV infection *even when they live* in households where there are *no* chronic carriers. These children are probably infected by playing with other children who are HBsAg infected from other households.[8] In addition, transmission of HBV in the household of a chronic carrier is most likely to occur between siblings when one sibling is the chronic carrier; in other words, horizontal transmission is more frequent than parent to child or child to parent.[9]

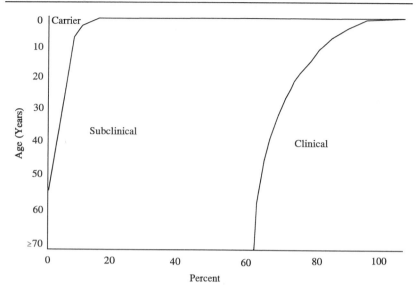

Figure 6.1 The relationship between age and outcome after acute HBV infection. Used with permission. Hollinger FB. Hepatitis B virus.In: Hollinger FB, Robinson WS, Purcell RH, et al, eds. *Viral Hepatitis*. New York: Raven Press, 1991: 73–138

Papular acrodermatitis is a skin manifestation (Gianotti-Crosti syndrome) of acute HBV in children (Figures 6.2A, 6.2B). In an epidemic of 153 cases in Japan, patients ranged from three months of age to ten years old.[10] Skin eruptions are the first sign of disease and are flat, erythematous and non-pruritic. They appear symmetrically on the face, buttocks and limbs; the trunk and mucous membranes are usually spared. The eruption evolves over several days and lasts one to four weeks. Lymphadenopathy involving the inguinal and axillary areas exists for two to three months.

HBsAg is detected early in most cases, but a few children will be seronegative initially and eventually develop anti-HBs. The acute hepatitis is usually mild and anicteric but aminotransferases may reach 1,000 to 2,000 IU/L. Immune complexes have not been identified in skin biopsies and Gionotti postulates this disorder is the clinical manifestation of primary natural infection with HBV acquired via mucous membranes or the skin.[11]

Limited data exists on the natural history of unselected childhood carriers of HBV. A New Zealand study achieved a greater than 90% testing of all children in a contained geographical area with 398 HBV carriers being discovered.[12] 15% were thought to perinatally acquired and the rest from childhood acquisition. Seroconversion of HBeAg+ to

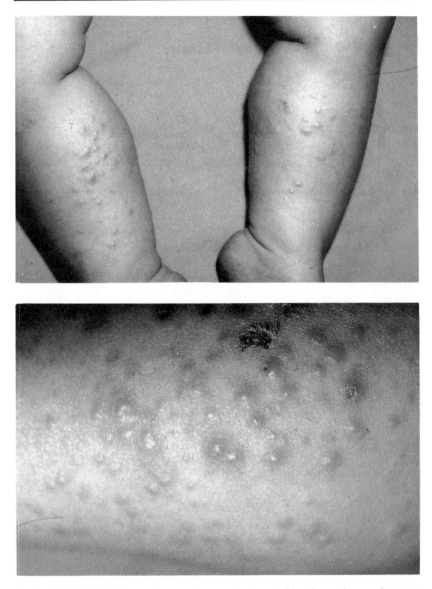

Figure 6.2A, B Multiple rounded papules occuring in a child with papular acrodermatitis (Gianotti-Crosti syndrome.) Photo courtesy of Dr. Kenneth Greer, University of Virginia Department of Dermatology.

HBeAg⁻ status occurred at a rate of 10.6% per year (figure 6.3). None of the children lost HBsAg. Only 22% and 7% of carriers showed an elevated and >2× normal ALT, respectively, at any time during the

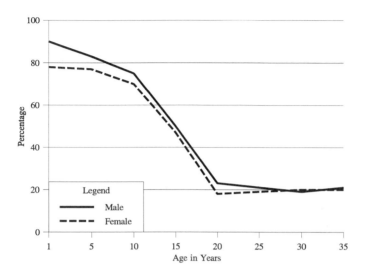

Figure 6.3 HBeAg by age and sex in HBV carriers. Used with permission. Moyes CD, et al. Liver function of hepatitis B carriers in childhood. *Pediatr Infect Dis J.* 1993; 12, issue 2, 120–125.

follow-up of 24 to 51 months. One child developed symptoms of hepatitis during this study and required referral to a specialist; in this case, symptoms resolved without specific treatment.

The disappearance of *e* antigen in children is an important event. In an Italian study, patients who lost *e* antigen also lost HBV-DNA and greatly downgraded their histological activity on liver biopsy.[13] Of 20 patients with chronic active hepatitis, 11 normalized their histology and nine regressed to chronic persistent hepatitis (CPH). Of eight with CPH, four normalized and four remained the same. A Japanese study noted similar clinical and histological improvement or resolution of liver disease with seroconversion of the *e* antigen. Clearance of the surface antigen[12–14] seldom occurs in childhood, but this is not unexpected since it may take ten to twenty years to clear the surface antigen after loss of the *e* antigen (Chapter 6). Reactivation of the *e* antigen, a common event in adults, is rarely reported in children.[12–14]

Whether a chronic carrier of HBV who acquires disease as a child fares better than a child who has been infected since birth is difficult to determine. A large unselected perinatally acquired HBV group has not been reported; studies with a selection bias do not appear to give a qualitatively different outcome from childhood acquired disease.[12–15]

In contrast to adults, liver biopsy in children appears to be much less valuable. The histology is usually minimal or normal[16] but even if chronic active hepatitis is present, it seldom progresses to cirrhosis. In a one to ten year follow-up of 166 Italian children with CAH due to HBV, none developed cirrhosis.[17] Of the ten children with HBV discovered to have cirrhosis, six had a second infection; either delta (3) or non-A, non-B hepatitis (3) present.[17] Only one of these ten children with cirrhosis developed decompensated liver disease after nine years of observation, this child was infected with both HBV and delta agent.[17]

Alfa-interferon (IFN) for treatment of chronic hepatitis B is reviewed in Chapter four. At the current time, the Food and Drug Administration in the United States has approved alfa-interferon 2b for use in patients over age 18. Few studies exist concerning the treatment of hepatitis B with alfa-interferon in children (Chapter 8). Available data suggests that carrier children should not be routinely treated with alfa-interferon.[18,19]

Finally, the development of hepatocellular carcinoma (HCC) occurs very rarely in the pediatric age group. As mentioned in Chapter 5, screening for HCC with ultrasound or alfa-fetoprotein has little utility and is not recommended for adult or pediatric patients.

HBV in adolescents

Adolescents, ages 11–19, constitute nine percent of acute hepatitis B cases reported to the CDC. Sexual transmission appears to be an important factor in this age group since cases begin to occur after the onset of sexual activity. Risk of infection is associated with a positive serologic test for syphilis and the number of sexual partners reported.[20]

Difficult Serology

The generalizations about hepatitis B serological markers given in Chapter four are intended for didactic purposes. The following material explains uncommon serological profiles which are confusing.

Isolated hepatitis B core IgG antibody

In a series of 700 asymptomatic federal prisoners tested by RIA, 3% were found to have an isolated core antibody (unpublished, Bader, Kibby). Smaller studies have noted a 0.5% to 20% rate of isolated core antibody by RIA testing.[21]

In the presence of a clinical picture of acute viral hepatitis, the core antibody in either the IgG or IgM form may be the only marker during the *window* period. However, in the asymptomatic patient with near normal aminotransferase levels and an undetectable anti-HBs antibody, acute hepatitis B is unlikely.

There can be multiple interpretations. An IgG isolated core antibody may indicate in order of likelihood: (1) a false positive antibody; (2) evidence of prior infection; or (3) chronic infection with HBV with an undetectable HBsAg. Ordering an IgM anti- HBc antibody will *not* help to distinguish between these possibilities.

The finding of an isolated core antibody has become more common since most laboratories have switched from RIA methodology to enzyme (EIA) testing. With EIA testing, the marker is more often false-positive.[22] 60% of patients with isolated IgG antibody given the vaccine respond with low levels of surface antibody indicating a primary or de novo exposure to HBV antigen.[23] A primary vaccination response in this situation means that the isolated IgG antibody is a false-positive result.

The HBV surface antibody lasts for a shorter period of time than the core antibody so a few patients with remote infection will present with only a core antibody. Up to 10% of patients who resolve acute HBV will never form surface antibody. 35% of patients with an isolated IgG core antibody by EIA will respond with a high titer of anti-HBs level consistent with an anamnestic response. An anamnestic response indicates prior infection and current immunity.[23]

The third possibility is that the patient has a low level HBsAg infectious titer. Donor units of blood containing only the anti-HBc marker have rarely transmitted HBV.[21]

MacIntyre's finding of two(6%) patients with isolated core antibody not responding to HBV vaccine could be interpreted as the presence of a chronic infection. RIA and EIA testing of the surface antigen are of comparable sensitivity but only detect down to 10,000,000 surface antigen particles per ml of blood. These results can be further defined with a more sensitive assay called HBV DNA. Detection of HBV DNA in serum by molecular hybridization is positive with as few as 5,000 to 10,000 molecules of HBV DNA (~0.05 pg).[24] MacIntyre's two patients were tested for HBV DNA and were negative.[23] Others, however, have rarely obtained a positive result with HBV DNA in this situation. Silva, et al. found a positive HBV-DNA result in one of 109 patients with isolated core antibody by EIA.[22]

The concern about an isolated core antibody is heightened when it is discovered in a serological workup for an asymptomatic transaminase elevation. For practical purposes, an isolated core antibody is irrelevant in this clinical situation. In the rare case where the core antibody may be the only marker of low level infection, it is not contributing to the current hepatic injury since damage tends to be proportional to circulating levels of the virus.

There is no proof that transmission of HBV has occurred from a HBsAg-negative, anti-HBc IgG positive patient in any setting except through blood transfusions. Further, these patients are not hazards to the blood supply since they are now excluded by anti-HBc donor testing.

For the foregoing reasons, at our institution, we exclude the anti-HBc IgG antibody from the "chronic hepatitis profile" ordered by physicians to evaluate occult liver disease. IgG anti-HBc testing is useful for screening blood donors, and in instances when indicated, pre-testing for the need of HBV vaccine. IgM anti-HBc and HBsAg are the serological markers of choice to evaluate acute viral hepatitis due to HBV (Chapter 4).

Isolated hepatitis B surface antibody

Anti-HBs is the only serological marker to develop after HBV vaccination. Outside of vaccination, the finding of this antibody alone is unusual. In the study of 700 prisoners screened for HBV markers referred to previously, none had an isolated anti-HBs marker. Other smaller studies have shown a rate of 0–7% by RIA testing.[21]

The finding of an isolated anti-HBs without prior vaccination or known disease is a peculiar finding in health care workers. Kessler, et al, report that 36% of nonvaccinated health care workers with at least one marker for HBV have isolated anti-HBs.[25] Employees with this serological profile are thought not to be protected from future infections. HBV vaccine given in this situation produces an anamnestic response in 25% of recipients suggesting only a minority of people with isolated anti-HBs are protected.

Coexistent surface antigen and surface antibody

Rare cases are encountered where the surface antibody and surface antigen are both positive. Simultaneous occurrence of these markers to form immune complexes occurs in conditions such as the arthritis-dermatitis syndrome.[18] The surface antibody in these instances is usually not detected because it is absorbed by the large excess of surface antigen present. Coexistence of these markers can occur, however, without any definable immune complex disease taking place.[24]

It is possible that the patient has been infected with two different strains of HBV and the antibody is reacting to one.[26] Regardless, these patients are considered infectious.

Coinfection with Hepatitis B and Human Immunodeficiency Virus (HIV)

Coinfection with HBV and HIV is common since both have similar epidemiologic patterns. In a group of 233 HIV positive subjects in San Francisco, 11% were chronically infected with both viruses.[27]

Influence of HIV upon HBV infection

Long term followup of homosexual men who participated in the large hepatitis B vaccine trial from 1980 provides valuable data on the effects of HIV upon HBV infection. In non-vaccinated HIV carriers who were acutely infected with HBV, 21% became chronically infected with HBV compared to a 7% rate in those men who were HIV- negative.[28] The rate of chronic infection appears even worse in asymptomatic HIV positive drug addicts who are acutely infected with HBV; in one study, 89% became chronic carriers of HBV compared to a 2% carrier rate if the addict was HIV-negative.[29]

Cell-mediated immunity plays a central role in the pathogenesis of HBV. Hepatitis B virus does not appear to be cytopathic to hepatocytes. In practical terms, this means HBV does not cause liver damage by itself. Damage of "hepatitis" occurs when the immune system, in the form of cytotoxic T-lymphocytes and other cells, attacks infected hepatocytes. Impairment of the cell mediated system, as in HIV disease, is likely to modify the course of HBV infection with less hepatocyte damage (i.e. hepatitis).

A number of clinical observations support the concept that HIV infection modifies HBV infection. In acute hepatitis B, the peak alanine aminotransferase (ALT) values are found to be similar in both HIV positive and negative groups; but, in 12 to 36 month followup, those with HIV infection have lower ALT levels.[28] The histological picture in HIV coinfection is less severe with reduced fibrosis when compared to HIV negative HBV carriers.[30]

HIV-positive subjects who clear HBV have higher helper T-lymphocyte counts (mean 547×10^6/L) than those who become carriers of HBV (mean $352 \times 10^6/L$).[31] Coinfected HBV carriers are unlikely to clear HBV when interferon is prescribed.[32]

The author has yet to see an HIV infected patient die from hepatitis B disease alone. Hepatitis B tends to be a minor issue compared to other clinical problems in these unfortunate patients.

Influence of HBV upon HIV infection

For HBV to have a direct influence on HIV infection, it must infect the same cells. HBV is predominantly a hepatotropic virus but HBV-related DNA has been found in lymphoid cells and T-lymphocytes. A reduction in helper T-lymphocytes has been found in one study of chronic HBV carriers who are HIV-negative. A reduced helper T-lymphocyte population should theoretically accelerate the progression of HIV-disease since the helper T-cell is the target of the HIV virus; however, large epidemiological studies do not suggest that progression to AIDS is more rapid in HBV carriers.[28]

Even when AIDS is established, a four year followup study does not demonstrate any difference in survival[27] (Figure 6.4) Thus, HBV appears to have little or no effect on the clinical course of HIV infection.

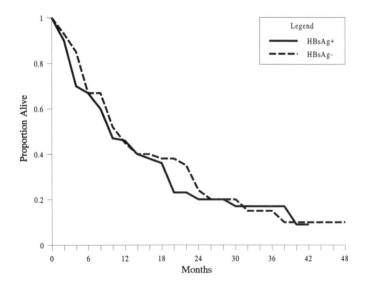

Figure 6.4 Twenty-four HBsAg-positive and 48 HBsAg-negative patients with an established diagnosis of AIDS. Reproduced with permission from Scharschmidt B, et al. Hepatitis B in patients with HIV infection: relationship to AIDS and patient survival. *Ann Intern Med* 1992; 117:837–838.

References

1. Rawal BK, Parida S, Watkins R, et al. Symptomatic reactivation of hepatitis B in preganancy. *Lancet* 1991; 337:364.

2. Chan G, Yeoh E, Young B, et al. Effect of pregnancy on the hepatitis B carrier state. In: Lemon SM, Margolis H, eds. *Viral hepatitis and liver disease: proceedings of the 1990 International symposium on Viral Hepatitis and Liver Disease.* Baltimore: Williams and Wilkins, 1991:678–680.

3. Hieber J, Dalton D, Shorey J, et al. Hepatitis and pregnancy. *J Pediatrics* 1977; 91:545–549.

4. Rustgi VK. Cirrhosis and pregnancy. Ini Rustgi VK, Cooper JN, eds. *Gastrointestinal and hepatic complications in pregnancy.* New York: John Wiley, 1986:200–216.

5. Boxall E, Flewett T, Dane D, et al. Hepatitis B surface antigen in breast milk. *Lancet* 1974; 2:1007–1008.

6. Beasley R, Stevens C, Shiao I, et al. Evidence against breast-feeding as a mechanism for vertical transmission of hepatitis B. *Lancet* 1975; 2:740–741.

7. Polito C, Manna A, Cartiglia M, et al. Normal growth of children with HBsAg positive chronic active hepatitis. *Acta Paediatri Scand* 1991; 80:1231–1232.

8. Franks A, Berg C, Kane M, et al. Hepatitis B virus infection among children born in the United States to Southeast Asian refugees. *N Engl J Med*; 1989; 321:130–135.

9. Craxi A, Tine F, Vinci M, et al. Transmission of hepatitis B and hepatitis delta viruses in the households of chronic hepatitis B surface antigen carriers: a regression analysis of indicators of risk. *Am J Epid* 1991; 134:641–649.

10. Toda G, Ishimaru Y, Mayumi M, et al. Infantile papular acrodermatitis (Gianotti's disease) and intrafamilial occurrence of acute hepatitis B with jaundice: age dependency of clinical manifestations of hepatitis B virus infection. *J Inf Dis* 1978; 138:211–216.

11. Seeff LB. Diagnosis, therapy, and prognosis of viral hepatitis. In: Zakim D, Boyer TD, eds. *Hepatology: a textbook of liver disease.* Philadelphia: WB Saunders, 1990.

12. Moyes CD, Milne A, Waldon J, et al. Liver function of hepatitis B carriers in childhood. *Pediatr Infect Dis J* 1993; 12:120–125.

13. Sodeyama T, Kiyosawa K, Akahane Y, et al. Evolution of HBeAb/Anti-HBe status and its relationship to clinical and histological outcome in chronic HBV carriers in childhood. *Am J Gastroenterology* 1986; 81:239–245.

14. Bortolotti F, Cadrobbi P, Crivellara C, et al. Long-term outcome of chronic type B hepatitis in patients who acquire hepatitis B virus infection in childhood. *Gastroenterology* 1990; 99:805–810.

15. Lok AS, Lai CL, Wu PC, et al. Spontaneous hepatitis B e antigen to antibody seroconversion and reversion in Chinese patients with chronic hepatitis B virus infection. *Gastroenterology* 1987; 92:1839–1843.

16. Chang M, Hwang L, Hsu H, et al. Prospective study of asymptomatic HBsAg carrier children infected in the perinatal period: Clinical and liver histologic studies. *Hepatology* 1988; 8:374—377.

17. Bortolotti F, Calzia R, Cadrobbi P, et al. Liver cirrhosis associated with chronic hepatitis B virus infection in childhood. *J Ped* 1986; 108:224–227.

18. McMahon BJ. What should we clinicians do for healthy, asymptomatic, HBsAg-positive carriers? *Hepatology* 1993; 18:1014–1016.

19. Koff RS. Hepatitis B today: Clinical and diagnostic overview. *Pediatr Infect Dis J* 1993; 12:428–432.

20. Margolis HS, Alter MJ, Hadler SC. Hepatitis B: evolving epidemiology and implications for control. *Sem Liver Dis* 1991;11:84–92.

21. Hoofnagle JH, Seeff LB, Bales ZB, et al. Serologic responses in hepatitis B. In: Vyas GN, Cohen SN, Schmid R, eds. *Viral Hepatitis*. Philadelphia: Franklin Institute Press, 1978:219–242.

22. Silva AEB, McMahon BJ, Parkinson AJ, et al. HBV DNA by PCR in individuals with anti-HBc as the only marker of hepatitis B virus infection. *Hepatology* 1992; 16:65 (abstract).

23. McIntyre A, Nimmo G, Wood G. Isolated hepatitis B core antibody—can response to hepatitis B vaccine help elucidate the cause? *Aust NZ J Med* 1992; 22:19–22.

24. Shafritz DA, Sherman M, Tur-kaspa R. Hepatitis B virus persistence, chronic liver disease and primary liver cancer. In: Zakim D, Boyer TD, eds. *Hepatology: a textbook of liver disease*. Philadelphia: WB Saunders, 1990:945–957.

25. Kessler HA, Harris AA, Prayne JA, et al. Antibodies to hepatitis B surface antigen as the sole hepatitis B marker in hospital personnel. *Ann Intern Med* 1985; 103:21–26.

26. Koziol DE, Alter HJ, Kirchner JP, et al. The development of HBsAg-positive hepatitis despite the previous existence of antibody to HBsAg. *J Immunology* 1976; 117:2260–2262.

27. Scharschmidt B, Held M, Hollander H, et al. Hepatitis B in patients with HIV infection: relationship to AIDS and patient survival. *Ann Intern Med* 1992; 117:837–838.

28. McNair A, Main J, Thomas H, et al. Interactions of the human immundeficiency virus and the hepatotropic virus. *Sem Liver Dis* 1992; 12:188–196.

29. Monno L, Angarano G, La Caputo S, et al. Unfavorable outcome of acute hepatitis B in anti-HIV-positive drug addicts. In: Zuckerman AJ, ed. *Viral Hepatitis and Liver Disease.* New York: Alan Liss, 1988:205–206.

30. Bodsworth N, Cooper D, Donovan B. The influence of human immunodeficiency virus type 1 infection on the development of the hepatitis B virus carrier state. *J Infect Dis* 1991; 163:1138–1140.

31. Goldin R, Fish D, Hay A, et al. Histological and immunohisto-chemical study of hepatitis B virus in human immunodeficiency virus infection. *J Clin Pathol* 1990; 43:203–205.

32. McDonald J, Caruso L, Karayiannis P, et al. Diminished responsiveness of male homosexual chronic hepatitis B virus carriers with HTLV-III antibodies to recombinant alfa-interferon. *Hepatology* 1987; 7:719–723.

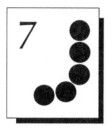

Prevention of Hepatitis B

Hepatitis B Vaccine
Safety
Hepatitis B Immunoglobulin
Universal Vaccination of Children
High Risk Groups
Post-Exposure Treatment
Non-Responders
Are Boosters Necessary?

Hepatitis B virus (HBV) infection is a global problem. Over 300 million chronic carriers of HBV exist worldwide and 1.5 million of these carriers reside in the United States. An estimated 200,000 to 300,000 acute infections with HBV occur annually in the United States. The Centers for Disease Control estimates that HBV has infected up to 12,000 health care workers (HCW) annually. 300 of these HCW die each year. To contrast with AIDS, no HCW have died from AIDS contracted on the job; yet, disproportionate concern continues to focus on the HIV virus.[1] The risk of HBV infection is 100x that of HIV infection after needlestick. A mathematical model predicts the risk of death for dentists from occupationally acquired HBV infection exceeds that of HIV by a factor of 1.7.[2] The tragedy is HCW continue to die from an infection preventable by a safe vaccine.

The strategy of restricting the hepatitis B vaccine to groups at high risk of contracting infection has failed to impact the incidence of hepatitis B. Acute cases of hepatitis B reported yearly in the United States have diminished significantly in recent years but not as a result of the use of the hepatitis B vaccine (Figure 7.1). The first decline in the incidence curve for cases of hepatitis B from 1985 to 1988 took place as a result of changes in high risk behavior in homosexuals.[3] Since 1989, the decline has been due to a 40% reduction in the incidence of hepatitis B cases among injection drug users, possibly as a result of safer needle-using practices.[3]

The reason for the limited impact of the vaccine is that it has been given sparingly. Many cases of hepatitis B cannot be prevented with a restricted policy since half of new hepatitis B cases in the United States occur in persons who are not members of identified high risk groups. Inasmuch as only 50% of HCW have accepted the hepatitis B vaccine, it is doubtful that any other high risk group will achieve a better vaccination status. Recent Occupational, Safety and Health rules enacted in the United States require all HCW to accept the hepatitis B vaccine or sign a refusal form; these rules should improve acceptance and awareness about the vaccine.[4]

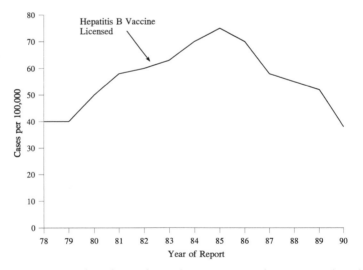

Figure 7.1 Estimated incidence of acute hepatitis B, United States, 1978 through 1990. The decline from 1985 to 1988 was due to a marked decrease in the incidence in homosexuals. The decline from 1989 was due to a decrease rate in intravenous drug users since rates in homosexuals have been stable since 1989 (CDC).

The Immunization Practices Advisory Committee (ACIP) now recommends universal childhood vaccination starting at time of delivery or during routine health care visits.[5]

Hepatitis B Vaccine

The first hepatitis B vaccine used in the United States was derived from plasma donors with extremely high levels of hepatitis B surface antigen. A double blind trial in 1,083 homosexual men gave a protective rate of nearly 100%. The vaccine prevented acute hepatitis B, asymptomatic infection, and chronic antigenemia. 95% of vaccinated subjects developed antibody against the surface antigen.[6] The plasma derived vaccine is no longer available in the United States. Irrational ideas about transmitting AIDS and higher production costs were factors in discontinuing production. Given the intense purification and inactivation process, concerns about any disease being transmitted with the vaccine were never justified.[7]

Vaccines are now produced by recombinant DNA technology. The recombinant vaccines use synthetic hepatitis B surface antigen (HBsAg) (an incomplete virus particle) created by inserting a gene for HBsAg into *Saccharomyces cerevisiae* (common baker's yeast). HBsAg is purified by lysing the yeast cells and separating the surface antigen from yeast components. Two yeast recombinant vaccines are available in the United States (Figure 7.1). Recombivax-HB (Merck, Sharpe and Dohme) and Engerix-B (Smith-Kline Biologicals) are both safe and effective in a variety of clinical situations.[8, 9] Figure 7.2 reviews doses for different patient populations. Figure 7.4 illustrates the long-term protection of adult responders to hepatitis B vaccine.

Table 7.1 Characteristics of HBV vaccines produced in the United States.

	Plasma* Derived	Yeast-Recombinant	
Manufacturer	MSD	MSD	SKB
Trade name	Hepavax®	Recombivax HB®	Engerix-B®
HBsAg protein/ml	20 µg	10 µg	20 µg
HBsAg glycosylated	Yes	No	No
Chemical treatment	Pepsin, uread formaldehyde	Formaldyhyde	None

*The plasma derived vaccine is no longer available. MSD=Merck, Sharpe, and Dohme. SKB = Smith, Kline Biologicals.

Table 7.2 Recommended doses of currently licensed hepatitis B vaccines (CDC1).

Group	Recombivax HB		Energix-B	
	Dose (μg)	(ml)	Dose (mg)	(ml)
Infants of HBsAg-negative mothers and children < 11 years	2.5	(0.5)[1]	10	(0.5)
Infants of HBsAg-positive mothers; prevention of perinatal infection	5	(0.5)	10	(0.5)
Children and adolescents 11–19 years	5	(0.5)	20	(1.0)
Adults ≥ 20 years	10	(1.0)	20	(1.0)
Dialysis patients and other immunocompromised persons	40	(1.0)[2]	40	(2.0)[3]

Both vaccines are routinely administered in a three-dose series. Engerix-B has also been licensed for a four-dose series administered at 0, 1, 2, and 12 months.

[1]New pediatric formulation (MMWR, September 10, 1993, p. 687).

[2]Special formulation.

[3]Two 1.0 ml doses administered at one site, in a four-dose schedule at 0, 1, 2, and 6 months.

Table 7.3 Long-term protection among adult responders to hepatitis B vaccine.

Long-term Protection Among Adult Responders to Hepatitis B Vaccine					
Study group	Years of follow-up	Number	Anti-HBs < 10 m IU/ml(%)	Anti-HBc positive (%)	HBV carriers number
Homosexual men	8	634	(54)	(7)	0
Homosexual men	10	127	(42)	(4)	0
Alaskan natives	10	262	(27)	(1)	0
Health care workers	5	174	(24)	(0)	0

Data derived from:
    Viral Hepatitis and Liver Disease, Baltimore: Williams & Wilkins; 1991:766–8
    Pediatrics 1993; 90:170-3JAMA 1989; 261:2362–6; CDC, unpublished data
    Viral Hepatitis and Liver Disease, New York: Alan P. Liss; 1988:998–1001   CDC

Safety

The hepatitis B vaccines have been more thoroughly evaluated and intensively monitored than any vaccine in the history of medicine. Over four million adults in the United States are vaccinated and at least that many children have received the vaccine worldwide.

In placebo controlled studies, side effects of the hepatitis B vaccine are less than placebo for all symptoms; the only exception being pain at the injection site. In various trials, temporary pain at the injection site occurs 3–29%. Among children receiving both hepatitis B vaccine and DTP vaccine, side effects are no more frequent than among children receiving DTP vaccine alone.[10]

Reports show a few cases of Guillain-Barré (GBS) in adults receiving the plasma derived vaccine. An extremely low rate of 0.5/100,000 vaccinees coincidentally occurred and this incidence is *far lower* than would be expected in a comparable non-vaccinated, age matched population.[7] Similarly, no association of GBS has been noted with use of recombinant vaccines in over 2.5 million recipients.[10]

Erythema nodosum after vaccination is rare;[11] since this benign dermatologic condition occurs in natural infection with HBV (Chapter 4), the observation is probably valid.

Thus, it is clear that the hepatitis B vaccines are entirely safe.[12] Any theoretical risk of a tiny and presumed side effect must be balanced against the expected risk of acute and chronic liver disease from hepatitis B during life. There is at least a 5% lifetime risk of acquiring HBV infection in the United States. For each U. S. birth cohort (children born each year), 2,000 to 5,000 persons will eventually die from HBV-related liver disease.[10]

Hepatitis B Immunoglobulin

Hyperimmune hepatitis B immunoglobulin (HBIG) is a plasma derived product containing a high titer of anti-HBs. HBIG has an anti-HBs titer of > 100,000 compared to < 1,256 in regular immune serum globulin. Plasma used for HBIG is screened for antibodies to HIV. The Cohn fractionation process inactivates and eliminates HIV from the final HBIG product. There is no evidence that HIV can be transmitted by HBIG.[10, 13]

HBIG is a useful adjunct to the administration of hepatitis B vaccine in babies born to HBsAg positive mothers and in sexual contacts. HBIG does not inactivate or blunt the immune response to hepatitis B vaccine when administered at the same setting but in different injection sites.

A detailed review of trials involving HBIG is written by Leonard Seeff.[13]

Universal Vaccination of Children

Infants born to HBsAg-negative mothers

The ACIP recommends all infants receive the hepatitis B vaccine.[5] It is given separately or simultaneously in a different muscle site with other vaccines. Hepatitis B vaccine can be given intramuscularly in the antero lateral thigh or upper arms at all ages, including birth. The buttock site should not be used since lower immunogenicity from this site occurs in adults and because the sciatic nerve can be injured.[14] The hepatitis B vaccine does not come mixed with other childhood vaccines; however, mixed vaccines should be available in the future. The hepatitis B vaccine, when given in different sites, is compatible with all other childhood vaccines.[5, 14]

Table 7.4 presents recommended schedules of hepatitis B vaccine for infants born to HBsAg negative mothers. A three-dose schedule is necessary. The first dose is given at birth or within the first two months of life. Increasing the interval beyond two months for the second dose has little effect on antibody levels. The third dose is *necessary* for optimal protection and acts as a booster. The third dose should be separated by at least two months from the second; but, higher antibody levels are achieved if the third injection is given at least four months

Table 7.4 Recommended schedules of hepatitis B vaccination for infants born to HBsAg-negative mother (CDC).

Hepatitis B Vaccine	Age of Infant
	Option One
Dose 1	Birth—before hospital discharge
Dose 2	1–2 months
Dose 3	6–18 months
	Option Two
Dose 1	1–2 months
Dose 2	4 months
Dose 3	6–18 months

after the second. The third dose works well if given up to one year after the second.

Infants born to HBsAg-positive mothers

Table 7.5 outlines the vaccination approach and HBIG use in an infant born to a HBsAg positive mother. All women should be routinely tested for HBsAg during an early prenatal visit; in addition, those pregnant women at high risk of HBV infection (e.g. intravenous drug abusers or those who develop intercurrent sexually transmitted disease) should have their HBsAg tested again before delivery.[10]

Table 7.5 Recommended schedule of hepatitis B immunoprophylaxis to prevent perinatal transmission of hepatitis B virus infection (CDC).[4]

Infant Born to Mother Known to Be HBsAg Positive	
Vaccine dose[†]	*Age of infant*
First	Birth (within 12 hours)
HBIG[§]	Birth (within 12 hours)
Second	1 month
Third	6 months*

Infant Born to Mother Not Screened for HBsAg	
*Vaccine dose*****	*Age of infant*
First	Birth (within 12 hours)
HBIG[§]	If mother is found to be HBsAg positive, administer dose to infant as soon as possible, not later than 1 week after birth
Second	1–2 months[††]
Third	6 months*

[†]See Table 7.2 for appropriate vaccine dose.

[§]Hepatitis B immune globulin (HBIG)—0.5 ml administered intramuscularly at a site different from that used for vaccine.

*If four-dose schedule (Engerix-B) is used, the third dose is administered at 2 months of age and the fourth dose at 12–18 months.

**First dose = dose for infant of HBsAg-positive mother (see Table 7.2). If mother is found to be HBsAg positive, continue that dose; if mother is found to be HBsAg negative, use appropriate dose from Table 7.2.

[††]Infants of women who are HBsAg negative can be vaccinated at 2 months of age.

Women admitted for delivery who have not had prenatal HBsAg testing should have blood drawn as soon as possible for testing. While test results are pending, the infant should receive hepatitis B vaccine within 12 hours of birth. The dose should be the same as for infants born to a *HBsAg-positive* mother (Tables 7.2 and 7.5). If the mother is found to be HBsAg-positive, her infant should receive HBIG as soon as possible and within seven days of birth. If HBIG is not administered, the second dose of vaccine must be given at one month and not later than two months of age because of the high risk of infection.[5, 10]

HBIG or hepatitis B vaccine given alone to an infant born to a mother who is both HBsAg and HBeAg positive appear to have only a 70–75% protection rate. The combination of HBIG and vaccine in-

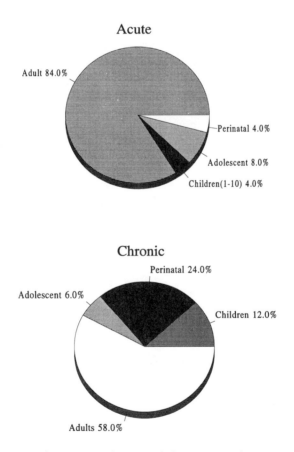

Figure 7.2 Age of acquisition of acute and chronic HBV infections. United States, 1989 estimates (CDC).

creases the protection rate to 90–95% but 5–10% of infants still become infected.[13]

Pregnancy

Pregnancy or lactation are not contraindications to receiving the hepatitis B vaccine. No fetal damage occurs.[10] This should be expected since natural infection with HBV during pregnancy does not cause congenital defects (Chapter 6).

Issues Concerning Universal Vaccination of Infants

Objections to universal vaccination consist of cost, low disease occurrence in children and acceptability.[15, 16]

The cost of the three dose vaccine series, excluding the office visit, in adults is about $100. The cost of the series for an infant born to a HBsAg negative mother ranges from $21 in the public sector to $28 in the private sector. Cost savings occur when vaccination begins in neonates rather than waiting until adolescence. The vaccine dose in infants is one-half that of adolescents. Physician visits are scheduled for newborn care, whereas, the cost of three separate physician visits for teenagers would be incurred. In addition, short of mandatory law, adolescents are unlikely to comply with a vaccine series.

Over the next few years, universal vaccination of infants will prevent a minority of acute hepatitis B cases (8%) that occur in the United States. However, since infants have a much higher rate of developing chronicity than adults (Chapter 6), perinatal and childhood acquisition accounts for 36% of chronic carriers in the United States (Figure 7.2).

The child born to a HBsAg-negative family has a 5% risk of acquiring the disease during his or her lifetime. The incidence varies in U.S. population groups, but by 30 years of age, 3–25% of any population group will encounter HBV infection. This prevalence is much greater than for any other disease now being prevented by immunization.[17] In terms of morbidity and mortality, hepatitis B represents a greater disease burden than any other vaccine preventable disease in history (Table 7.6).

Acceptance of the vaccine by parents depends on the enthusiasm of the health care provider. Asking the parent if they want their child vaccinated against the most common chronic infectious disease and the most common cause of liver cancer in the world will produce a favorable response. On the other hand, if the provider fails to present a clear rationale or exhibits worry about the extra shot, an unfavorable atti-

Table 7.6 Estimated lifetime morbidity and mortality of vaccine preventable diseases before availability of vaccines (CDC).

Estimated Lifetime Morbidity and Mortality of Vaccine Preventable Diseases Before Availability of Vaccines

Disease	Clinical cases (per million)	Long-term sequelae (per million)	Deaths (per million)
Hepatitis B	25,000	7000	1000–1500
H. influenza b invasive disease	5,000	1500	300–600
Measles	900,000	300	200–400
Mumps	75,000	5	3–5
Polio	14,000	4500	100–400
Pertussis	600,000	40	200–300
Rubella	300,000	750	10–15

tude from the parent can be expected. The current generation of parents are too young to remember the ravages of the last disease, polio, which is nearly extinct due to vaccination. The generation 20 years or older at the introduction of the polio vaccine in the 1950's eagerly accepted any new vaccine. Subsequent age groups, because of a lack of direct observation of epidemic diseases, need more education by health care professionals.

Since the introduction of the vaccine in 1982, the chief objection to utilization has been cost. Safety and efficacy are not issues. However, the cost per dose of hepatitis B vaccine is similar to that of other recommended childhood vaccines.[18] Cost-effectiveness of routine infant vaccination compares favorably to other medical interventions (Table 7.7). Again, the problem for American medicine is the focus on life-saving, expensive and dramatic procedures to save lives rather than on prevention.[19] The relevant example is liver transplantation for cirrhosis due to hepatitis B. Such an operation costs about 225,000 dollars and 10,000 dollars per year to maintain the recipient. Such costs might be worthwhile if long-term survival were excellent, but as reviewed in chapter eight, the one year survival after transplantation is 50%–60%. For our health care organization, avoidance of one such transplant per year would easily fund the costs of the infant vaccination program for hepatitis B and much of the cost of vaccinating all adolescents.

Table 7.7 Cost-effectiveness of selected medical interventions 1992, U.S. Dollars (CDC).

Cost-Effectiveness of Selected Medical Interventions 1992, U. S. Dollars	
Intervention	*Cost per year of life saved*
Routine infant hepatitis B vaccination	$1,852
Antepartum administration of anti-Rh immune globulin	2,329
Smoking cessation—nicotine gum	7,450
Neonatal intensive care (1000–1400 g infants)	7,987
Coronary artery bypass surgery (left main disease)	10,595
Pneumococcal vaccination (>65 years of age)	11,456

Transplantation for hepatitis B related disease is considered experimental by many transplant centers. Nonetheless, failure to refer such a patient for transplantation can result in expensive litigation. In the author's opinion, health organizations who demonstrate a high vaccine compliance rate in children and adolescents should be protected by law from litigation involving failure to transplant for hepatitis B.

The American Academy of Pediatrics recommends vaccination of all adolescents when resources permit.[17] Implementing a universal approach now in adolescents would cause a more rapid decline in hepatitis B disease. Short of vaccinating the entire population, the policy of selecting vaccination for high-risk adult groups is necessary. Unfortunately, such a policy has a low awareness and compliance rate among health care professionals.

Preexposure Vaccination

Susceptibility testing

High risk groups are outlined in Table 7.8. Prevaccination serologic testing is cost-effective in groups with a HBV marker prevalence of >20%.[20] For routine testing (to avoid vaccine administration), anti-HBc is the most common marker present in high risk groups since it is present in both chronic carriers and immune individuals; however, anti-HBc does not differentiate between these two groups. Only one antibody needs to be measured. Anti-HBs testing will identify immune

Table 7.8 Prevalence of hepatitis B serologic markers in various population groups. Groups are listed in order discussed in text (modified from CDC[1]).

Population group	Prevalence of Serologic Markers of HBV Infection	
	HBsAg%	Any marker (%)
Household contacts of HBV carriers	3–6	30–60
Health-care workers—frequent blood contact	1–2	15–30
Patients of hemodialysis units	3–10	20–80
Sexually active homosexual men	6	35–80
Heterosexuals with multiple partners	0–5	5–20
Prisoners	1–8	10–80
Clients in institutions for the developmentally disabled	10–20	35–80
Immigrants/refugees from areas of high HBV endemicity	13	70–85
Users of illicit parenteral drugs	7	60–80

individuals but not chronic carriers (Chapter 4).[6] False positivity is *extremely low* in members of *high-risk* groups.

Pretesting for HBV markers in a low risk population is not necessary. Hepatitis B vaccine produces neither a therapeutic nor adverse effect on HBV carriers. Those who are immune from prior infection will experience an increase in their anti-HBs levels.

Household contacts

Household contacts of a chronic carrier are the most frequently missed high risk group. When HBV carriers are identified through blood donor, prenatal or other routine screening, their household and sexual contacts should be tested for possible vaccination. Office or school contacts need not be vaccinated.

Medical care

Health care workers (HCW) in contact with patients or blood are strongly encouraged to receive the vaccine. Susceptible hemodialysis patients need vaccination with a larger than usual dose (Table 7.2). Identification of patients early in the course of their renal disease is helpful since higher seroconversion rates and antibody levels are achieved in patients vaccinated before the need for dialysis.[21]

Patients who require repetitive blood transfusions or clotting-factor concentrates should be vaccinated as soon as their disorder is identified.

In the few HIV positive patients not already HBV marker positive, an initial vaccination series should be offered. If a poor response occurs, repeat vaccination will not improve the outcome.[22]

Sexual activity

Homosexual men and heterosexual men and women with multiple sexual partners are at increased risk of HBV infection. Methods of transmission are reviewed in Chapter 3. Identification of this group is difficult. If other sexually transmitted diseases occur, then vaccination is indicated. A sexual behavior history in the past year should be obtained from every adolescent or adult. Inquiring about a monogamous relationship is not sufficient, particularly in adolescents, since many patients are "monogamous" for several months at a time. " Serial monogamy" can be a reason to consider vaccination.

Condoms derived from natural sources can leak HBsAg under experimental conditions. Latex condoms do not leak HBsAg microscopically[23] but any condoms can rupture 1–8% of the time. Other body secretions, such as saliva, are potentially infectious;[24] thus, reliance on the use of condoms alone is not sufficient to prevent the transmission of HBV.

Since it is neutral in connotation, the preferred term is "sexually active" rather than "promiscuous." However, health care providers can appear so neutral about sexuality that the patient receives the impression that sexual activity is risk free. Reinforcement of abstinence or monogamous activity with an uninfected partner should be emphasized as the only completely "safe" way to avoid venereal disease or AIDS.

Institutional groups

Prisoners are a high risk group for HBV since many engage in IV drug abuse and homosexual activity. Early calculations suggested an incidence rate of 5–10% per year but seroconversion studies have shown a 1–2% rate. Nonetheless, this is far greater than the general population. Vaccination is desirable; however, funding for prisons is usually the lowest priority in government budgets. At the minimum, susceptible

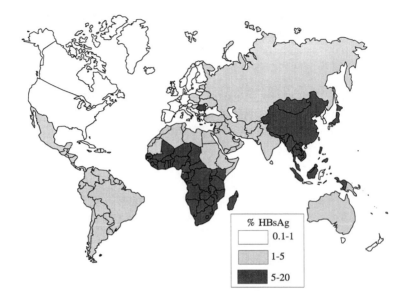

Figure 7.3 Prevalence of HBsAg around the world.

IV drug abusers and female prisoners should be vaccinated since these groups have been shown to have a high seroconversion rate in prison.[25]

Clients and staff of institutions for the developmentally disabled should be screened for susceptibility and vaccinated.[10]

Contact with endemic areas

Immigrants and adoptees from areas with a high rate of endemic disease (Figure 7.3) should be screened for HBV markers. If an HBsAg carrier is identified, all household contacts should be vaccinated. Even if a carrier is not found in an immigrant family from an endemic area, children < 7 years of age should be vaccinated since there is a high rate of interfamilial HBV infection (Chapter 6).

International travelers who plan to reside for more than six months in an HBV endemic area should be vaccinated. Short term travelers may be vaccinated if they plan to have blood or sexual contact in that area.[26] Areas and planned activities warranting vaccination are listed in Table 7.9.

Hepatitis B vaccination for travelers should begin six months before travel to allow complete vaccination. This is often not possible and a

Table 7.9 Areas and activities where travelers are recommended to receive the hepatitis B vaccine (CDC[25]).

Areas (HBV Carrier Prevalence > 5%)

- Sub-Sahran Africa
- Southeast Asia
- South Pacific Islands
- Interior Amazon Basin
- Parts of the Caribbean (Haiti, Dominican Republic)

Travel Description

- Residence > 6 months
- Short-term travel *which includes:*
  - > Health care work or exposure to blood
  - > Sexual contact with population

partial series will offer some protection. An alternative four dose schedule of injection at zero, one and two months will give fair protection with a 4th dose at 12 months for a booster effect.[10]

Intravenous drug abusers

Intravenous drug abusers (IVDA) are the highest risk group for acquiring hepatitis B. Vaccination is offered for the minority who are seronegative for HBV markers.

Post-Exposure Treatment

In an accidental percutaneous (needlestick, laceration, or bite) or mucosal (ocular or mucous membrane) exposure to blood, evaluation and treatment is based upon a number of factors: (1) whether the source of the contaminated blood is available (i.e. donor); (2) the HBsAg status of the source; and (3) the hepatitis B vaccination status of the recipient.

When possible, the donor of the body secretion needs to be identified and tested for HBsAg, anti-HCV and HIV markers (Table 7.10). The recipient, if previously vaccinated, should be tested for anti HBs. Anti-HBs need not be tested in the recipient if it is known to be positive within twenty-four months prior to the exposure incident. A person

Table 7.10   Evaluation of acute percutaneous or musosal exposure to blood

1. If possible, attempt to find source of blood (i.e. donor).
2. If available, test source for HBsAg, HIV antibody and anti-HCV.
3. Test recipient for anti-HBs (unless tested in prior 24 months), HIV antibody and anti-HCV.
4. If recipient anti-HBs negative, see Table 7.11 for treatment
5. If donor or recipient positive for HIV antibody, refer to local institutional protocol.
6. If donor or recipient positive for anti-HCV, refer to Chapters 10,11.

sustaining a significant exposure to blood should also have an HIV antibody and hepatitis C antibody (anti-HCV) drawn.

It is beyond the scope of this text to evaluate a positive HIV test in either the donor or recipient. The uncertain value of gamma globulin for recipients exposed to hepatitis C is reviewed in chapter eleven. Anti-HCV is drawn at the time of blood exposure to establish whether or not the recipient has been previously exposed or is a carrier to hepatitis C. In the author's experience, documentation of prior susceptibility or infection with hepatitis C is very helpful in workmen's compensation cases.

When information is gathered about the source and exposed person, Table 7.11 reviews recommendations from the CDC. If the physician evaluating the incident requests a rapid HBsAg and anti-HBs, these can usually be done within twenty-four hours (instead of four to seven days for a *routine* hepatitis B profile). For proven effectiveness, HBIG should be given as soon as possible after the exposure; the value of receiving HBIG after seven days is uncertain.

Post-Vaccination Testing

Hepatitis B vaccine given in the deltoid muscle to healthy persons produces a protective antibody (anti-HBs) in more than 90% of recipients. Testing for immunity after vaccination is not necessary except when subsequent management depends on knowing the immune status. Health care workers with significant occupational exposure to blood should have follow-up testing for adequate immunity—defined as anti-HBs levels mIU/ml.[5]

Infants born to HBsAg positive mothers should have their anti-HBs levels checked three to nine months after the completion of the vaccine series.[16]

All other groups should only undergo testing directly after a significant exposure to hepatitis B as outlined inTable 7.11.

Table 7.11 Recommendations for hepatitis B prophylaxis following percutaneous or permucosal exposure.

Exposed Person	Treatment When Source Is Found To Be:		Source Not Tested or Unknown
	HBsAg-positive	HBsAg-negative	
Unvaccinated	HBIG × 1* and initiate HB vaccine[†]	Initiate HB vaccine[†]	Initiate HB vaccine[†]
Previously vaccinated			
Known responder	Test exposed for anti-HBs 1. If adequate[§], no treatment 2. If inadequate, HB vaccine booster dose	No treatment	No treatment
Known nonresponder	HBIG × 2 or HBIG × 1 plus 1 dose HB vaccine	No treatment	If known high-risk source, *may treat as if source were HBsAg-positive*
Response unknown	Test exposed for anti-HBs 1. If inadequate[§], HBIG × 1 plus HB vaccine booster dose 2. If adequate, no treatment	No treatment	Test exposed for anti-HBs 1. If inadequate[§], HB vaccine booster dose 2. If adequate, no treatment

*HBIG dose 0.06 ml/kg IM

[†]HB vaccine dose—see Table 7.2

[§]Adequate anti-HBs is ≥ 10 SRU by RIA or positive by EIA

Non-Responders to Vaccination

About 5% of healthy, immunocompetent young adults fail to develop protective levels of anti-HBs with a series of three vaccine injections. The primary reason for non-response appears to be under genetic control. A major histocompatibility complex haplotype (HLA-B8, SCO1, DR3) has been identified and acts as a recessive trait. Helper T-cell function is necessary for adequate B-cell production of surface antibody.[27] Other conditions associated with poor response to the vaccine include gluteal injection, obesity, age over 60, and altered immunity.[5, 28, 29]

Revaccination of non-responders produces adequate antibody in 15 to 25% after one additional dose and 30–50% after three additional doses in the deltoid muscle.[10] Unfortunately, initial non-responders who later develop antibody lose their antibody much more quickly. In one study, a repeat three dose vaccination series produced a good response (> 10 RU) in 41% of subjects but only 8% of subjects retained this antibody level 18 months later. Poor responders to the initial vaccination series do better than non-responders with revaccination: 79% respond to the second series and 29% keep adequate levels of antibody 18 months later.[30] In comparison, nearly 100% of responders to the primary vaccination series retain a protective antibody level at 18 months.

Duration of Antibody Response: Are Boosters Necessary?

The degree of protection induced by the hepatitis B vaccine is dependent on a protective antibody response developing after vaccination. Antibody persistence correlates with peak levels achieved after the last vaccine dose. Antibody levels then decline steadily with time. In responding adults who are immunocompetent, many studies demonstrate detectable anti-HBs in 85% of subjects five years after vaccination; 60–80% of subjects have levels (> 10 mIU/ml) considered protective.[31]

Nonetheless, if a patient has an initial response to the vaccine (i.e. > 10 mIU/ml) and then loses detectable antibody, protection against clinically significant hepatitis B appears to continue for up to ten years (Table 7.3). Infections that occur after disappearance of antibody are asymptomatic and manifested only by the appearance of hepatitis B core antibody. In the large homosexual trial mentioned earlier, only one patient who responded to vaccine and then lost antibody had an overt infection manifested by the presence of HBsAg and aminotransferase greater then 2½ × normal. This patient was also HIV-infected and he did not (M. Alter, personal communication) become a chronic carrier.[30] 5-10 year follow-up of several populations (Table 7.3) have not demonstrated the development of a chronic carrier state in any vaccinated group despite loss of detectable antibody.

Booster doses are unnecessary for responders with a normal immune system for up to ten years after receiving the vaccine. The need for booster doses after more than ten years is being evaluated.

Hemodialysis patients require annual assessment of susceptible anti-HBs levels (< 10 mIU/ml) and revaccination when necessary.[10]

Vaccine Storage and Shipment

The vaccine should be shipped and store at 2–8°C but *not frozen*. *Freezing* destroys the potency of the vaccine.[10]

Conclusion

Health providers need better awareness of the magnitude of hepatitis B and more aggressiveness in identifying and vaccinating high risk groups. In the author's opinion, when resources permit, the hepatitis B vaccine should be offered to anyone under age fifty who desires it. Only an aggressive approach will make a significant impact on the most common chronic infectious disease in the world.

References

1. Goldsmith MF. Even in perspective, HIV specter haunts health care workers most. *JAMA* 1990; 263:2413–2420.
2. Krause DS. Hepatitis B in the emergency department. *N Engl J Med* 1992; 327:1032.
3. Alter MJ, Mast EE. The epidemiology of viral hepatitis in the United States. *Gastroenterology Clinics of North America* (in press).
4. OSHA stiffens bloodborne rules, decrees free hepatitis B vaccine. *Am J Nursing* 1992; Jan:82–84.
5. Centers for Disease Control: Hepatitis B virus: a comprehensive strategy for eliminating transmission in the United States through universal childhood vaccination. *MMWR* 1991; 40 (RR-13).
6. Szmuness W, Stevens CE, Zang EA, et al. A controlled clinical trial of the efficacy of the hepatitis B vaccine (heptavax B): a final report. *Hepatology* 1981; 1:377–385.
7. Bader TF. A protocol for needle-stick injuries. *Emer Med* 1986; 18:36–43.
8. Stevens CE, Taylor PE, Tong MJ, et al. Yeast-recombinant hepatitis B vaccine. *JAMA* 1987; 257:2612–2616.

9. Andre FE, Safary A. Clinical experience with a yeast-derived hepatitis B vaccine. In: Zuckerman AJ, ed. *Viral Hepatitis and Liver Disease*. New York: Alan Liss, 1988: 1025–1030.

10. Centers for Disease Control: Protection against viral hepatitis: Recommendations of the Immunization Practices Advisory Committee (ACIP). *MMWR* 1990; 39(S-2).

11. Goolsby PL. Erythema nodosum after Recombivax HB hepatitis B vaccine. *N Engl J Med* 1989; 321:1198–1199.

12. McMahon BJ, Helminiak C, Wainwright RB, et al. Frequency of adverse reactions to hepatitis B vaccine in 43,618 persons. *Am J Med* 1992; 92:254–256.

13. Seeff L. Diagnosis, therapy and prognosis of viral hepatitis. In: Zakin D, Boyer TD, eds. *Hepatology*, Philadelphia: WB Saunders, 1990.

14. Committee on Infectious Diseases: Universal hepatitis B immunization. *Pediatrics* 1992; 89:795–800.

15. Farber JM. Hepatitis B immunization. *Pediatrics* 1992; 89:981-2.

16. Some concern over instituting hepatitis B vaccine into babies' routine vaccination schedules. *Inf Control Hosp Epid* 1991; 12:745–746.

17. Hall, C. Hepatitis B immunization: in reply. *Pediatrics* 1992; 89:982.

18. Peter, G. Childhood immunizations. *N Engl J Med* 1992; 327:1794 and 1800.

19. Voelker R. Prevention ranks low in U. S. health care spending. *Amer Med News*. August 10, 1992:3.

20. Hashimoto F. Cost effectiveness of serotesting before hepatitis vaccination. *N Engl J Med* 1982; 307:503.

21. Seaworth B, Drucker J, Starling J, et al. Hepatitis B vaccines in patients with chronic renal failure before dialysis. *J Infect Dis* 1988; 157:332–337.

22. Hadler SC. Hepatitis B prevention and human immunodeficiency virus. *Ann Int Med* 1988; 109:92–94.

23. Minuk GY, Bohme CE, Bowen TJ, et al. Efficacy of commercial condoms in the prevention of hepatitis B virus infection. *Gastroenterology* 1987; 93:710–714.

24. Scott RM, Snitbhan R, Bancroft WH. Experimental transmission of hepatitis B virus by semen and saliva. *J Infect Dis* 1980; 142:67–71.

25. Bader TF. Hepatitis B in prisons. *Biomedicine and Pharmacotherapy* 1986; 40:248–251.

26. Centers for Disease Control. Health information for international travel 1990. *HHS publication no. 90-8280.*

27. Alper CA, Kruskall MS, Marcus-Bagley D, et al. Genetic prediction of nonresponse to hepatitis B vaccine. *N Engl J Med* 1989; 321:708–712.

28. Weber DJ, Tutala WA, Samsa GP, et al. Obesity as a predictor of poor antibody response to hepatitis B plasma vaccine. *JAMA* 1985; 254:3187–3189.

29. Denis F, Mounier M, Hessel L, et al. Hepatitis B vaccination in the elderly. *J Inf Dis* 1984; 149:1019.

30. Hadler SC, Francis DP, Maynard JE, et al. Long-term immunogenicity and efficacy of hepatitis B vaccine in homosexual men. *N Engl J Med* 1986; 315:209–214.

31. Gibas A, Watkins E, Hinkle C, et al. Long-term persistence of protective antibody after hepatitis B vaccination of healthy adults. In: Zuckerman AJ, ed. *Viral Hepatitis and Liver Disease.* New York: Alan Liss, 1988: 998–1001.

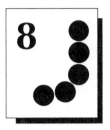

Treatment of Hepatitis B

Alfa-Interferon Therapy
Liver Transplantation

Alfa-Interferon Therapy

Hepatitis B virus can cause progressive liver disease and cirrhosis in as many as 25% of adult chronic carriers. The approval of alfa-interferon 2b for treatment of chronic hepatitis B in adult patients by the United States Food and Drug Administration in 1992 represents the first effective therapy available.

Hepatitis B virus (HBV) and Hepatitis C virus (HCV) respond very differently to treatment with alfa-interferon. The treatment of hepatitis C is reviewed in Chapter 9.

HCV and HBV cause liver injury in dissimilar ways: HCV causes direct injury to the hepatocyte by itself and is considered a cytopathic virus; HBV, in contrast, is not directly injurious to liver cells; liver injury occurs due to a cytotoxic attack from the host's immune system.[1] Thus, the degree of injury in HBV (i.e. hepatitis) depends on the response of the immune system.

The response to alfa-interferon also illustrates the difference in cytopathic response. Treatment with alfa-interferon in HCV causes a diminuation of aminotransferase values, such as the ALT, and thus an amelioration in the degree of hepatitis. When HCV is inhibited, less

117

direct damage occurs. In contrast, alfa-interferon treatment of HBV causes an increase in ALT values (i.e. flare) or worsening of hepatitis. 63% of HBV patients treated will experience a flare of hepatitis during alfa-interferon therapy (defined as > 2 × baseline ALT value).[2] Occasionally, the flare can be severe in patients with advanced liver disease, causing decompensation or death.

The molecular biology of cellular damage is more complex than cytopathic (HCV) vs non-cytopathic (HBV); however, the distinction will help the clinician understand why alfa-interferon lessens hepatitis due to HCV and often worsens the hepatitis due to HBV. Further, disease due to HBV can also be worsened with corticosteroids or chemotherapy agents whereas the disease caused by HCV is little affected by these agents.

Higher doses of alfa-interferon are required in treatment of HBV compared to HCV. Since side-effects are dose-related, the HBV patients will have more untoward reactions than HCV patients.

Thus, since hepatitis C is improved by alfa-interferon therapy a dedicated primary care physician may treat such patients. However, the author has three reasons to suggest that HBV patients should be treated only by liver specialists. One, the serology of HBV is complex; two, the flare that often occurs in HBV patients may cause an adverse event such as variceal bleeding or ascites; three, the dosage of alfa-interferon is higher and the side effects will be greater and require more experience in management.

Alfa-interferon and the immune system interferons are a class of proteins produced by mammalian cells with a wide spectrum of antiviral, antiproliferative and immunomodulatory effects (Table 12.2). Monocytes and lymphocytes make alpha-interferon in response to viral and antigenic stimuli. After cellular uptake, interferons induce proteins that mediate antiviral actions. A virus, by definition, cannot synthesize nucleic acids or proteins. It must take over the cellular mechanisms of the host cell to replicate (Figure 12.1). Alfa-interferon stimulates a protein called 2'5'-oligo-adenylate synthetase that appears to inhibit takeover of protein synthesis by the virus.

Invasion of a host cell by a virus results in expression of proteins onto the cell surface. Inhibition of these signals must occur for a virus to escape recognition by circulating lymphocytes and establish a persistent presence. Alfa-interferon appears to promote the surface expression of membrane proteins; these *marked* cells can then be destroyed by cytotoxic T-cells.[3]

Efficacy

The goal of alfa-interferon therapy for chronic hepatitis B is to permanently suppress or eliminate the virus and cause a remission of the associated liver disease.

HBV is thought to be suppressed by alfa-interferon when markers of active viral replication, such as *HBeAg* and *HBV DNA*, disappear. The virus is eliminated and the carrier state terminated when *HBsAg* is no longer present. Clearance of HBV surface antigen does not usually occur after initial alfa-interferon therapy and therapeutic trials have shown only a 10–20% resolution of HBsAg at the end of therapy. However, most, if not all, of patients who remain persistently HBeAg negative and HBV-DNA negative will eventually eliminate HBsAg (Figure 8.1).[4] Thus, when efficacy is cited, not only HBsAg outcome but HBeAg and HBV-DNA results are relevant.

16 randomized controlled trials with a total of 498 patients have been reported with alfa-interferon treatment administered for three to six months with follow-up for six to twelve months after therapy. The aggregate response rate is 37% of patients lose HBV-DNA, 33% lose HBeAg and 8% lose HBsAg.[5]

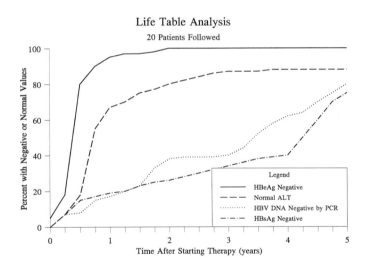

Figure 8.1 Serologic and biochemical values in 20 patients who had a long-term response to alpha-interferon therapy with percentage negative or normal values over time. The duration of treatment was 4 months in most patients. Time 0 = time of initiation of interferon therapy. HBeAg = hepatitis B e antigen; ALT = alanine aminotransferase; HBsAg = hepatitis B surface antigen; HBV DNA = hepatitis B virus DNA; PCR=polymerase chain reaction. Reproduced with permission, from Korenman J, et al. Long term remission of chronic hepatitis B after alpha-interferon therapy. *Ann Intern Med* 1991; 114:629–34.

Table 8.1 Categories of response to IFN. Data derived from Perrillo RP, et al. A randomized, controlled trial of interferon alfa-2b alone and after prednisone withdrawal for the treatment of chronic hepatitis B. *N Engl J Med.* 1990; 323:295–301.

	Categories of Response to IFN		
	Optimal *40–50%*	*Moderate* *20 - 30%*	*Poor* *0-5%*
HBV-DNA pg/ml	< 100	100-200	> 200
			or
ALT	> 200	100-200	< 100

However, a number of variables appear to predict treatment response. The U. S. trial, Hepatitis Interventional Therapy Group, identified pre-treatment ALT and HBV-DNA levels as important (Table 8.1). A high ALT value (> 200 IU/L) and low HBV-DNA level (< 100 pg/ml) appear very predictive of response.[6] In other words, a patient with an active immune system (i.e., high ALT) and low viral load suggests that an endogenous attempt to eliminate infected hepatocytes is already taking place. The latter patients appear to benefit most from alfa-interferon treatment.

Two other variables, HIV positivity and perinatal acquisition are negative predictors for treatment response (Table 8.2). HIV positive patients uniformly fail to respond to alfa-interferon.[7,8] Co-infected HIV and HBsAg patients have very high HBV-DNA levels and low ALT values (Chapter 6).

Ethnic Chinese patients have a much lower response rate to alfa-interferon.[9,10] Some have thought this is related to long duration of infection associated with perinatal infection. However, Chinese children also respond poorly to alfa-interferon suggesting the low response rate is not due to delayed treatment.[9] Others have reported a

Table 8.2 Patient variables and response to alfa-interferon therapy.

Positive Response	Negative Response
Low pre-therapy HBV-DNA	High pre-therapy HBV-DNA
High pre-therapy ALT	Low pre-therapy HBV-ALT
Active histology	HIV positive
	Perinatal acquisition
	Delta positive

higher antibody level to alfa-interferon (presumably blocking the therapeutic effect) in Oriental patients.[11]

Again, most Chinese patients have high HBV-DNA levels and normal ALT values, a situation referred to as "immune tolerance" and this is probably what is causing their poor response rather than ethnic origin. The response of perinatally acquired HBV to alfa-interferon in African or Caucasian patients has not been reported.

When Chinese patients are selected for an elevated ALT value (mean of three pretreatment levels > 1.5 × normal), their response rate, 15/39, 38%, does not appear different from reports in Western countries. The response rate in the normal ALT Chinese group was essentially zero.[9]

Other pretreatment variables such as active histology (positive response) and the presence of delta hepatitis (negative response) are probably also explainable by the host-virus interaction.

Table 8.3 Adverse conditions as percentages reported for the two standard dosage regimens used in hepatitis B. Hematologic reductions are listed in Table 8.4. Data derived from Intron A.® *Physicians Desk Reference.* Medical Economics, Montvale, NJ ©1994.

	Alfa-Interferon Dose	
Adverse experience	5 million IU QD	10 million IU tiw
Early		
Fever	66	86
Headache	61	44
Myalgia	59	40
Fatigue	75	69
Late		
Diarrhea	19	8
Anorexia	43	53
Nausea	50	33
Depression	17	6
Irritability	16	12
Alopecia	26	38

Adverse effects of alfa-interferon

Adverse effects of alfa-interferon are common and occur in a dose-dependent fashion. The doses for treatment of hepatitis B, 5 million units daily or 10 million units thrice weekly, are much higher than for hepatitis C (3 million units thrice weekly); thus, the clinician treating hepatitis B will encounter more toxicity from alfa-interferon.

The side-effects (Tables 8.3 and 8.4) appear either early (first few doses) or late (after one to two weeks). For the most part, the early symptoms are "influenza-like" and usually subside after the first few doses. Acetaminophen given in regular doses can help ameliorate symptoms. Fatigue is the most prominent symptom throughout therapy and tends to abate as interferon is continued.[12] Patients can usually continue to work and should be encouraged to do so. Management of various symptoms that may arise during alfa-inferferon therapy is reviewed in Table 8.5.

A side-effect of alfa-interferon which occurs to some degree in all HBV patients is myelosuppression. Table 8.4 shows that of patients who begin therapy with normal hematologic values, only a few experience severe changes. However, in the patient who has diminished values before therapy, usually due to hypersplenism and cirrhosis, the reduction in blood counts can be dramatic and life-threatening (see later section on treatment of cirrhosis).

Depression and irritability can be major problems in 6–17% of patients.[2] In the author's experience, patients with a prior history of major

Table 8.4 Abnormal hematological values versus dosage of alfa-interferon. It should be appreciated that patients began treatment with normal hematologic values. The below experience does not relate to patients who begin with low values due to hypersplenism and cirrhosis. Data derived from Intron A®. *Physicians Desk Reference*. Medical Economics, Montvale, NJ ©1994.

Abnormal Hematological Values Versus Dosage of Alfa-Interferon			
Laboratory test	Change	5 million IU QD (%)	10 million IU tiw (%)
Hemoglobin	$\geq 2mg/dl$	32	23
White blood cell count	$< 3,000/mm^3$	68	34
Granulocyte count	$1,000-1,500/mm^3$	30	32
	$750-1,000/mm^3$	24	18
	$500-750/mm^3$	17	9
	$< 500/mm^3$	4	2
Platelet count	$<70,000/mm^3$	12	5

Table 8.5 Management of symptomatic side-effects during alfa-interferon use.

> **Influenza-type reaction** – acetaminophen or ibuprofen prn. Reaction usually disappears after the second injection.

> **Malaise** – diphenhydramine prn. Emphasize liberal fluid intake and mild exercise.

> **Nausea, anorexia** – cisapride (10 mg PO QID) may help.[13] Interferon dose may need to be reduced (Table 8.8).

> **Depression, irritability** – a tricyclic anti-depressant, fluoxetine and/or co-management by psychiatrist may be needed.

> **Fever** – occurring within the first two weeks of treatment may be secondary to starting alfa-interferon. It should respond to acetaminophen or ibuprofen. After two weeks, any fever should have an immediate medical evaluation to exclude serious bacterial infection.

depression are most likely to suffer this side-effect. If the patient has had major psychiatric problems in the past, alfa-interferon therapy may even be contraindicated; at the least, such a patient should be co-managed with a psychiatrist.[14] The author has also found it helpful to have the patient's spouse present at the pre-treatment counseling session so they can be forewarned about irritability.

The development of autoantibodies, with or without autoimmune disease, occurs in more than 50% of patients treated with alfa-interferon.[15] Fortunately, development of autoimmune disease is rare. Thyroid problems head the list of autoimmune disorders which may occur during alfa-interferon therapy and are quite uncommon; in clinical trials for treatment of hepatitis C, <1% (4/426) developed either hypothyroidism or hyperthyroidism.[2] The incidence of thyroid problems during treatment of hepatitis B appears to be much less than during treatment for hepatitis C.[16] Systemic lupus erythematosus, pernicious anemia, vasculitis, autoimmune thrombocytopenia and polyarthropathy have all been reported to occur in conjunction with alfa-interferon therapy.[12] Thus, until more is known, alfa-interferon therapy should be used with caution, if at all, in patients with a pre-existing autoimmune disorder.

Mild alopecia and diarrhea can occur and will resolve after the end of therapy. A few patients may have an acceleration of their male pattern of baldness.[17]

Bacterial infections are a serious adverse event. Cases of septicemia, lung abscess, brain abscess and bacterial peritonitis are reported. Cirrhotics, who already have significant humoral immunity defects, are particularly predisposed. Any fever occurring after the first two weeks of therapy deserves an immediate evaluation. The clinician should have a low threshold to start antibiotics early.[17]

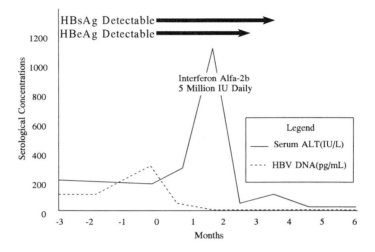

Figure 8.2 Example of a flare of ALT on alfa-interferon therapy.

Flare of hepatitis

A common reaction in patients who ultimately eliminate the hepatitis B virus is to have their ALT and bilirubin values rise mildly or dramatically during therapy. This is referred to as a "flare" of hepatitis and occurs from 4–16 weeks after initiation of therapy (Figure 8.2). It often occurs in conjunction with the disappearance of the "e" antigen. It is considered a "good" sign since 75% of those patients who respond to alfa-interferon flare during therapy. However, a flare is not necessary

---

Table 8.6 Management of hepatitis B flare with IFN.

Increase of ALT, bilirubin—symptomatic or asymptomatic

- Occurs 4–16 weeks (mean 8 weeks)
- More frequent monitoring needed (weekly or biweekly)
- Stop IFN if :
  - > Signs of decompensation
    - — Ascites
    - — Encephalopathy
    - — Variceal bleeding
  - > Severe laboratory changes
    - — Bilirubin > 4.0 mg/dl (68 μmol/L)
    - — Albumin < 2.7 g/dl

or predictive of an ultimate response since 25% of responders do not flare and 15% of patients who flare do not make a sustained response (data on file, Schering-Plough Corporation).

The flare is well tolerated in patients with adequate hepatic reserve[18,19] but deaths in patients with poor liver status before treatment are reported[6,20] (see treatment of cirrhosis).

The management of a flare is outlined in Table.6 8. Alfa-interferon should be discontinued if decompensation (i.e., appearance of ascites, bleeding or encephalopathy) occurs or significant hyperbilirubinemia or hypoalbuminemia develops.

Monitoring

Table 8.7 reviews the recommended laboratory monitoring for HBV patients. A dose reduction is needed in about 40% of patients receiving 5 million units daily.[12] Table 8.8 lists parameters for dose reduction or cessation of therapy (even if a flare does not occur). Fatigue and nausea may be incapacitating. Severe granulocytopenia and thrombocytopenia require stopping therapy. Despite the plethora of adverse symptoms, only 5% of patients treated with 5 million units daily have had to stop alfa-interferon therapy. Similar rates of dose modification and drop-outs have been reported in patients treated with 10 million units thrice weekly.[12]

Table 8.7 Monitoring for hepatitis B.

Monitoring for Hepatitis B

- Weeks 1, 2, and then monthly
  - > CBC, platelets, ALT, albumin, bilirubin
- Week 16 and 3, 6 months post-therapy
  - > HBeAg, HBsAg, ALT

Table 8.8 Alfa-Interferon dose reduction selection.

	Routine	Nausea	Granulocytes	Platelets × 1000
50% Reduction	Interference with daily routine	Daily nausea if unresponsive to cisapride	< 750/mm^3	< 50/mm^3
STOP	Bedrest	Vomiting > 2× daily	< 500/mm^3	< 30/mm^3

The two dosage regimens, 5 million units daily and 10 million units thrice weekly, appear to have similar efficacy and adverse profiles. The author favors the 10 million unit schedule since a smaller (and less expensive) total weekly dose of 30 million units is used. The recommended duration of treatment is 16 weeks.[2]

Patient selection

Inclusion

The approach to patient selection is based upon an understanding of factors which predict response and adverse effects of alfa-interferon. Table 8.9 lists criteria for a patient with a highly predictive (i.e., >75%) response to alfa-interferon. ALT levels and HBV-DNA levels are the most important pre-test values (Table 8.1).

HBV patients with normal ALT values or < 1.5× normal have nearly a zero response rate. Treatment of these patients will only waste money and make the patient temporarily sick to no avail. Disease due to HBV, however, is a dynamic situation. Patients with near normal ALT should be rechecked every six to twelve months. If the patient has a significantly elevated ALT at a later date, treatment can be started at that time.

While liver histology is not a selection factor, most authorities would recommend a liver biopsy before treatment. It is valuable in identifying the asymptomatic Child's class A cirrhotic who might tend to experience more difficulty with decompensation during therapy.

Table 8.9 Selection factors for hepatitis B treatment.

- \> 18 years old
- Chronic hepatitis—HBsAg$^+$ > 6 months
- HBeAg positive
- ALT > 100
- Low HBV-DNA level (< 100 pg/ml)
- Compensated liver disease
  > No history of encephalopathy, varices, ascites
  > Bilirubin normal
  > Albumin normal
  > PT Time < 3 secs prolonged
- WBC ≥ 4,000 /mm^3
- Platelets ≥ 100,000 /mm^3

Exclusion

Table 8.10 lists factors which should be considered to exclude patients. Some of the reasons, such as acute hepatitis B, are listed because of a lack of response to treatment; in others, such as significant cardiopulmonary disease, alfa-interferon can cause a deterioration due to fever and resultant tachycardia.

Active psychiatric problems are a contraindication to therapy. A past history of psychiatric problems remains a judgement for the clinician; certainly, if alfa-interferon is elected, patients with a significant past psychiatric history should be seen regularly by a psychiatrist during therapy.

Children

In the author's opinion, the purpose of treating children with chronic hepatitis B would be to change the natural history of the disease or to clear the infection entirely. Neither of these goals has been convincingly demonstrated.

Childhood carriers of HBV almost never develop cirrhosis prior to adulthood. This is true in both Caucasian and Oriental populations.[21-22] Even the rare finding of chronic active hepatitis does not appear ominous. An Italian study followed 166 pediatric patients with this pathologic lesion for one to ten years without any of the children developing cirrhosis.[21]

Three small trials have examined alfa-interferon treatment in young HBV carriers. 24 Chinese children were randomized to treatment with 10 million units/m² thrice weekly for 12 weeks or no treatment with no difference in outcome between the treated and control group.[25]

A follow-up study by the same Chinese group looked at prednisone or placebo pretreatment followed by 16 weeks of alfa-interferon.

Table 8.10 Conditions which should not be treated.

Do NOT Treat These Conditions with IFN:

- Acute hepatitis B or C
- "Healthy" carrier
- Decompensated liver disease (B virus)
- Children under 18 years of age
- Psychiatric history (relative)
- Immunocompromised patients
- Significant cardiopulmonary disease
- Transplant patients

Again, there was no statistical difference (at p < .05) between any treatment although there was a suggestion of response in the prednisone and alfa-interferon group of loss of HBV-DNA (16%) and e-seroconversion of 12.9%.[26]

A Spanish trial of 10 million units/m^2 thrice weekly for six months produced 50% response rate, as defined by loss of HBV-DNA, in the treated group and a 17% response rate in controls. Most children who lose HBV-DNA also lose e antigen.[27] However, in contrast to adults, no child lost HBsAg on follow-up several years later and HBV-DNA is still detected in all treated children by the more sensitive methodology, polymerase chain reaction.[28]

Thus, neither disappearance of infectivity nor change in natural history has been demonstrated in children with chronic HBV treated with alfa-interferon.

Larger trials are in progress now and may provide more information. At the current time, it is the author's contention that treatment of children with alfa-interferon should only be done in the context of a bona-fide clinical trial.

Cirrhosis and HBV infection

Unfortunately, some patients with HBV present for the first time with manifestations of decompensated cirrhosis such as persistent jaundice or variceal hemorrhage.

The National Institutes of Health has reported alfa-interferon treatment of 18 such patients.[20] Twelve patients initially responded to lower than standard doses of alfa-interferon with clearance of HBV-DNA. However, six of the responders relapsed with reappearance of HBV-DNA within 14 months after therapy. The six sustained responders had marked improvements in bilirubin and albumin values into normal range. All of the sustained responders became HBeAg negative and four cleared surface antigen. Side effects during therapy for cirrhosis due to HBV included bacterial infection (5), flare of hepatitis (9), psychiatric problems (3) and these problems led to stopping therapy in four, two, and three patients, respectively.

A large multicenter trial is now underway looking at low dose alfa-interferon for cirrhotics.[29]

Obviously, treatment of cirrhotics should be done only by an interested liver specialist. The possibility of severe reactions, including death, needs to be discussed with the patient.

Transplantation for End-Stage Liver Disease Due to Hepatitis B

In contrast to hepatitis C, the outcome of patients with chronic hepatitis B treated with transplantation is much poorer. The recurrence of infection in the new graft is nearly universal[30] and often leads to an accelerated disease culminating in advanced cirrhosis in as early as seven months and the *de novo* development of hepatocellular carcinoma in less than two years.[31] The one year and five year survival rates of patients after transplantation for chronic hepatitis B are 60% and 50% respectively, figures that are much poorer than for any other liver transplantation category except cancer.[30,32]

The risk of recurrence and the development of accelerated disease are clearly influenced by pre-transplant factors. The key predictor appears to be the pre-transplant load of virus and the degree to which the B virus is replicating.[33] Those patients who have evidence of active replication (HBeAg+ or HBV-DNA+) uniformly experience a recurrence of infection. In contrast, those patients who are HBV-DNA negative beforehand, recur in a range of 28 to 81%.[33]

The recurrence rates of hepatitis B are also lesser if the patient has fulminant hepatitis or co-infection with delta virus. A large European trial, with varying amounts of immunoprophylaxis, found a five year recurrence rate of 18% in fulminant hepatitis and a five year recurrence rate of 33% in delta/hepatitis B patients.[34] The ameliorating effect in fulminant hepatitis B appears to be the aggressive response of the immune system; while in delta hepatitis, the delta virus suppresses the replication of hepatitis B.

The return of accelerated disease due to hepatitis B produces a peculiar pathological pattern referred to as *fibrosing cholestatic hepatitis* (FCH).[35] Liver tests in these patients show markedly abnormal serum bilirubin and prothrombin times with only modest increases in serum aminotransferase levels.[36] When FCH occurs, it is uniformly fatal since the syndrome will recur in a second transplanted liver even more rapidly and cause death in less than seven weeks.[37]

Attempts have made to decrease the reinfection rate with peri-operative and post-operative administration of hyperimmune globulin specific for hepatitis B (HBIG). Results have been disappointing when HBIG is given for less than six to twelve months.[33,38] The utilization of long-term doses of HBIG has been hampered by cost (seven to fifteen thousand dollars per year) and the lack of approved formulation for intravenous administration for HBIG in the United States.[39] More work remains with long-term trials of HBIG after transplantation for tis B before an adequate answer is available. At best, current data seems to show that HBIG merely delays the time of recurrence of HBV rather than eliminating it.

Efforts have been made to decrease the recurrence of hepatitis B after transplantation with alfa-interferon but limited studies with a small number of patients have been unrewarding.[33] The fear of organ rejection has been the principle limiting factor in this situation. However, efforts with alfa-interferon in decompensated cirrhotics awaiting transplantation have yielded a significant proportion of patients who respond dramatically with clearance of the virus and enough return of liver function to resume an active life. Treatment of such cases must be limited to an experienced hepatologist since this approach can also worsen liver failure.

The outcome of transplantation for end-stage liver disease caused by HBV is so poor that Medicare, many insurance carriers and transplant centers consider the existence of actively replicating HBV to be a contraindication to transplantation.[39]

The costs of transplantation for liver disease are more expensive than for any other organ transplant. The median cost of hospitalization alone for a single patient in the United States in 1992 was $171,000 with total costs estimated at $225,000.[40] Each transplant requires $10,000 or more per year to maintain.

In contrast to transplantation, alfa-interferon 2b treatment for chronic hepatitis B (non-cirrhotic, e antigen positive) is clearly cost effective when compared to standard care.[41] In addition, a rational problem exists for developed countries which will cover transplantation costs for an individual but not pursue universal vaccination of the population (see also Chapter 7).

>> *As of this writing, a series of three hepatitis B immunizations for children in the United States cost $27.00. $225,000 for a transplant will provide 8,333 immunizations for children. The lifetime risk of acquiring acute hepatitis B is thought to be five percent with about five to ten percent of these developing the chronic carrier state. Thus, 416 acute infections and 20–42 chronic infections could be prevented with vaccination for the price of one liver transplant.*

Treatment Summary for Advanced Liver Disease Due to Hepatitis B

The survival outcome of advanced liver disease due to actively replicating hepatitis B appears to be about the same with alfa-interferon or transplantation; however, these approaches have never been compared in a randomized trial. Transplantation for liver disease due to actively replicating HBV should probably not be done outside the context of a bonafide clinical trial using HBIG immunoprophylaxis.

On the other hand, the few patients with fulminant hepatitis due to HBV or evidence of a low viral load (i.e., HBeAg⁻ or HBV-DNA⁻) do much better than those with active replication and would seem to be reasonable transplantation candidates.

The author favors low dose titration therapy for advanced liver disease rather than referral for transplantation. If financial resources of governments or insurance carriers are limited, they should be directed towards universal vaccination of infants and adolescents rather than transplantation for disease due to actively replicating HBV.

References

1. Maruyama T, Iino S, Koike K, et al. Serology of acute exacerbation in chronic hepatitis B virus infection. *Gastroenterology.* 1993; 105:1141–1151.

2. Intron® A. *Physician's Desk Reference*. Medical Economics Data. Montvale, NJ. 1995.

3. Peters M. Mechanisms of actions of interferons. *Sem Liver Dis* 1989; 9:235–239.

4. Korenman J, Baker B, Waggoner J, et al. Long-term remission of chronic hepatitis B after alpha-interferon therapy. *Ann Intern Med* 1991; 114:629–634.

5. Wong DK, Cheung AM, O'Rourke KO, et al. Effect of alpha-interferon treatment in patients with hepatitis B e antigen-positive chronic hepatitis B. *Ann Intern Med* 1993; 119:312–323.

6. Perrillo RP, Schiff ER, Davis GL, et al. A randomized, controlled trial of interferon alfa-2b alone and after prednisone withdrawal for the treatment of chronic hepatitis B. *N Eng J Med* 1990; 323:295–301.

7. Brook MG, McDonald JA, Karayiannis P, et al. Randomized controlled trial of interferon alfa 2A for the treatment of chronic hepatitis B virus infection: factors that influence response. *Gut* 1989; 30:1116–1122.

8. Brook MG, Chan G, Yap I, et al. Randomized controlled trial of lymphoblastoid interferon alfa in Europid men with chronic hepatitis B virus infection. *Br Med J* 1989; 299:652–656.

9. Lok AS, Wu PC, Lai CL, et al. A controlled trial of interferon with or without prednisone priming for chronic hepatitis B. *Gastroenterology* 1992; 102:2091–2097.

10. Lok AS, Lai CL, Wu PC, et al. Long-term follow-up in a randomized controlled trial of recombinant α-interferon in Chinese patients with chronic hepatitis B infection. *Lancet* 1988; 2:298–302.

11. Lok AS, Lai CL, Leung EK, et al. Interferon antibodies may negate the antiviral effects of recombinant α-interferon treatment in patients with chronic hepatitis B virus infection. *Hepatology* 1990; 12:1266–1270.

12. Perrillo RP. Interferon in the management of chronic hepatitis B. *Dig Dis Sci* 1993; 38:577–593.

13. Nishibayashi H, Kanayama S, Shinomura T, et al. Influence of interferon-alpha treatment on gastric emptying in patients with chronic hepatitis C. *Gastroenterology* 1995; 108:A657 (abstract).

14. Renault PF, Hoofnagle JH, Park Y, et al. Psychiatric complications of long-term interferon alfa therapy. *Arch Intern Med* 1987; 147:1577–1580.

15. Mayet WJ, Hess G, Gerken G, et al. Treatment of chronic type B hepatitis with recombinant α-interferon induces autoantibodies not specific for autoimmune chronic hepatitis. *Hepatology* 1989; 10:24–28.

16. Lisker-Melman M, DiBiscaglie AM, Usala SJ, et al. Development of thyroid disease during therapy of chronic viral hepatitis with interferon alfa. *Gastroenterology* 1992; 102:2155–2160.

17. Renault PF, Hoofnagle JH. Side effects of alpha interferon. *Sem Liver Disease* 1989; 9:273–277.

18. Hoofnagle JH, Peters M, Mullen KD, et al. Randomized, controlled trial of recombinant human α-interferon in patients with chronic hepatitis B. *Gastroenterology* 1988; 95:1318–1325.

19. Alexander GJ, Brahm J, Fagan EA, et al. Loss of HBsAg with interferon therapy in chronic hepatitis B virus infection. *Lancet* 1987; 2:66–68.

20. Hoofnagle JH, Di Bisceglie AM, Waggoner JG, et al. Interferon alfa for patients with clinically apparent cirrhosis due to chronic hepatitis B. *Gastroenterology* 1993; 104: 1116–1121.

21. Bortolotti F, Calzia R, Cadrobbi P, et al. Liver cirrhosis associated with chronic hepatitis B virus infection in childhood. *J Ped* 1986; 108:224–227.

22. Bortolotti F, Cadrobbi P, Crivellara C, et al. Long-term outcome of chronic type B hepatitis in patients who acquire hepatitis B virus infection in childhood. *Gastroenterology* 1990; 99:805–810.

23. Chang MH, Hwang LY, Hsu HC, et al. Prospective study of asymptomatic HBsAg carrier children infected in the perinatal period: clinical and liver histologic studies. *Hepatology* 1988; 8:374–377.

24. Sodeyama T, Kiyosawa K, Akahane, et al. Evolution of HBeAg/anti-HBe status and its relationship to clinical and histological outcome in chronic HBV carriers in childhood. *Am J Gastroenterology* 1986; 81:239–245.

25. Lai CL, Lok AS, Lin HJ, et al. Placebo-controlled trial of recombinant α-interferon in Chinese HBsAg-carrier children. *Lancet* 1987; 2:877–880.

26. Lai CL, Lau JN, Lok AS, et al. Effect of recombinant alpha interferon with or without prednisone in Chinese carrier children. *Quart J Med* 1991; 78:155–163.

27. Ruiz-Moreno M, Rua MJ, Molina J, et al. Prospective, randomized controlled trial of α-interferon in children with chronic hepatitis B. *Hepatology* 1991; 13:1035–1039.

28. Ruiz-Moreno M. Chronic hepatitis B in children: natural history and treatment. *J Hepatology* 1993; 17 (suppl 3):S64–66.

29. Perrillo R, Tamburro C, Regenstein F, et al. Treatment of decompensated chronic hepatitis B with a titratable, low dose regimen of recombinant interferon alfa 2-b. *Hepatology* 1992; 16:126A.

30. Starzl TE, Demetris AJ, Van Thiel D. Liver Transplantation. *N Engl J Med* 1989; 321:1092–1099.

31. Fagiuoli S, Shah G, Wright HI, et al. Types, causes, and therapies of hepatitis occurring in liver transplant recipients. *Dig Dis Sci* 1993; 38:449–456.

32. Gonzalez EM, Loinaz C, Garcia I, et al. Liver transplantation in chronic viral B and C hepatitis. *J Hepatology* 1993; 17 (Suppl 3): S116–S122.

33. Samuel D, Bismuth H. Liver transplantation for hepatitis B. *Gastroenterology Clinics of N. America* 1993; 22:271–283.

34. Samuel D, Muller R, Alexander G, et al. Liver transplantation in European patients with the hepatitis B surface antigen. *N Engl J Med* 1993; 329:1842–1847.

35. Davies SE, Portmann BC, O'Grady JG, et al. Hepatic histiological findings after transplantation for chronic hepatitis B virus infection, including a unique pattern of fibrosing cholestatic hepatitis. *Hepatology* 1991; 13:150–157.

36. O'Grady JG, Smith HM, Davies SE, et al. Hepatitis B virus reinfection after orthotopic liver transplantation. *J Hepatology* 1992; 14:104–111.
37. Wright T. The threat of hepatitis B virus recurrence: a sword of Damocles to the liver transplant recipient. *Hepatology* 1993; 18:219–222.
38. Mora NP, Klintmalm GB, Poplawski SS, et al. Recurrence of hepatitis B after liver transplantation: does hepatitis B immunoglobulin modify the recurrent disease? *Transplant Proceed* 1990; 22:1549–1550.
39. Perrillo RP, Mason AL. Hepatitis B and liver transplantation: problems and promises. *N Engl J Med 1993; 329:1885–1887.*
40. *Organ procurement costs highest for liver, study finds. Progress 1993;* 14:4 (published by American Liver Foundation, Cedar Grove, NJ 07009)
41. Wang JB, Koff RS, Tine F, et al. Cost-effectiveness of interferon-α2b treatment for hepatitis B e antigen-positive chronic hepatitis B. *Ann Intern Med* 1995; 122:664–675.

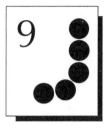

Diagnosis and Transmission of Hepatitis C

Discovery
Diagnostic Testing
Epidemiology and Transmission

Discovery

When serology for hepatitis A and B became available in 1974, the existence of a third hepatitis virus became apparent. Cases of acute hepatitis not associated with other diseases or drugs and that tested negative for hepatitis A and B were diagnosed as non-A, non-B hepatitis.

From 1978 to the mid-1980's, over 20 reports of specific antigen-antibody identification systems for the non-A, non-B virus appeared. In 1980, the National Institutes of Health submitted a coded panel of sera to laboratories around the world that claimed to have discovered an antigen or antibody to non-A, non-B hepatitis. On the coded panel were non-A, non-B sera verified as infectious by passage through chimpanzees. In addition, the panel contained sera from other liver diseases such as hepatitis B, primary biliary cirrhosis and alcoholic hepatitis. When the laboratories analyzed the coded panels, none could consistently identify the non-A, non-B sera and often identified

135

falsely the other liver diseases as positive for the non-A, non-B virus.[1] Despair prevailed in the 1980's, whether a reliable marker could ever be found for this disease.[2]

The principle reason for difficulty in identifying a marker for this virus is its very low concentration in serum. In contrast to hepatitis B, where the concentration of virus is one to ten million infective particles per ml of serum, only one to ten virions per ml of hepatitis C may be present.

Michael Houghton and colleagues, working at Chiron Corporation in California, adopted a new approach leading to success in 1989.[3, 4] Donor plasma with a high infectious titer was centrifuged into a pellet and the RNA from this pellet was extracted and through molecular biology techniques placed into the genome of *E. coli*. Clones were prepared and screened against non-A, non-B convalescent sera. After testing millions of clones, and six years hard work, a virus-specific clone was found which reacted with an antibody in the convalescent serum.

The c-100 assay, or what is now EIA-1, easily identified the coded NIH panels. The c-100 assay did not react with any of the sera from other liver diseases resulting in 100% specificity; however, it identified only 60% of the non-A, non-B (NANB) plasma on the panel. This was due to the fact that there were several acute NANB wells on the panel. Later investigation has shown the EIA-1 assay to have only a 10% sensitivity in acute hepatitis; however, if serial testing is done on acute NANB sera testing negative for EIA-1, as many as 80% of acute, post-transfusion NANB hepatitis will eventually seroconvert.

Since the discovery of a consistent marker for NANB hepatitis, the virus is now known as hepatitis C. EIA-1 testing is reviewed for historical purposes. The practical point of reviewing the development of the first enzyme linked assay for hepatitis C (HCV), is to remind the reader that EIA-1 became accepted on the basis of it's *specificity*; that is, it would not produce false-positive results when testing other liver diseases. So often, now, the writer hears physicians worry about false positive results with the anti-HCV test. False-positivity can occur in any diagnostic test when it is applied to a *low-risk* population (i.e., blood donors) but it is a minor concern when a patient with liver disease is tested.

Diagnostic Testing

To understand the sensitivity and specificity of HCV testing, various parts of its RNA genome and resulting antigens are illustrated in

Figure 9.1. In March 1992, Ortho Diagnostics introduced a second generation enzyme linked HCV test called EIA-2. The second generation system tests for two additional viral antigens, the C-22 and C-33 fragments (Figure 9.1). Antibodies to these latter antigens appear early. As a result, 50% of acutely infected HCV patients will test positive at the onset of symptoms and all patients become positive by 3-4 months after the onset of symptoms. Compared to EIA-1, EIA-2 detects HCV antibody 30 to 90 days earlier.[5] Depending on the definition of non-A, non-B hepatitis, as many as 90 to 95% of post-transfusion cases will test positive for HCV by EIA-2.0.[5, 6] Proportionately, EIA-2 detects 20 to 40% more cases of HCV than EIA-1.[5, 6]

A supplemental test approved by the FDA in 1993, RIBA-II, uses a different methodology to test for the same antigens as EIA-2 (Table 9.1). In addition to the c-100, c-33 and c-22 HCV antigens, RIBA-II detects a fourth antigen called 5-1-1 (Figure 9.1). Addition of the 5-1-1 antigen does not confer increased sensitivity,[6] but RIBA-II seems to clearly predict which questionable ELISA results are truly infectious.[7] The ability to predict infection is valuable in a low-risk population such as blood donors, who otherwise have a normal ALT and no signs of liver disease. RIBA-II positive blood donors can be referred for follow-up and possible treatment, while non-specific EIA positive and RIBA-II negative blood donors can be reentered into the donor pool.[7] However,

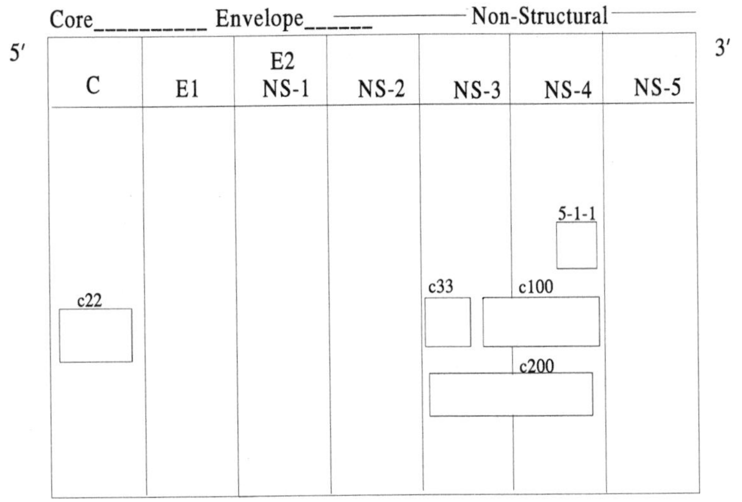

Figure 9.1 Structure of the HCV genome and associated viral proteins.

Table 9.1 Comparison of HCV tests. EIA-1 and RIBA-2 are obsolete. RIBA-4 is sometimes reported as RIBA-II to denote second generation but this can be confused with the first generation test referred to as RIBA-2 (denoting 2 antigens under test). This chapter will use the RIBA-II designation.

	Viral Antigens			
	c100	5-1-1	c33	c22
EIA-1	+	−	−	−
RIBA-2	+	+	−	−
EIA-2	+	−	+	+
RIBA-II (RIBA-4)	+	+	+	+

blood banks have not adopted a uniform policy for handling false-positive EIA-2 donors.

EIA-2 improves the specificity of testing in low-risk populations. Positive results of EIA-1 testing in blood donors, when verified with RIBA-II testing, show a 56% to 78% false positive rate.[8] In comparison, EIA-2 testing in the same setting has a 30% false positive rate.[9]

The approach to diagnosis depends on the patient population being evaluated. In a low risk population such as blood donors, who already have normal ALT values by definition, every positive EIA-2 test should be supplemented with a RIBA-II assay. The word "supplemental" is carefully chosen as a description of RIBA-II rather than "confirmatory" since the RIBA-II assay tests essentially the same viral antigens as EIA-2 but with a different approach. In a patient with evidence of liver disease, supplemental testing is not necessary if the patient has a clear risk factor for hepatitis C such as prior blood transfusion or intravenous drug use. Again, false-positivity is not a problem when applied to a high probability pre-test population.

Difficult serology

A problem with both EIA-2 and RIBA-II testing is the interpretation of a positive single band. Current methodology requires at least two bands (i.e., antigens) to be reactive before the EIA-2 or RIBA-II assay is called "positive." If only one band, such as the c-22 or c-33 fragment tests positive, the current approach is to label such a result "indeterminate."

A new technology called *polymerase chain reaction* (PCR) may help clarify diagnostic issues in hepatitis C. The PCR test multiplies minute quantities of genetic material such as RNA or DNA to a detectable level. In the case of hepatitis C, RNA is being multiplied. PCR can give a quantitative result concerning viral replication and infective presence that antibody tests cannot. For example, if the EIA-2 or RIBA-II assay is positive but PCR testing is negative, the probable interpretation is that the patient has cleared the infection and that the antibodies represent immunity. The other possibility is that the patient is having intermittent viremia.

In regard to indeterminate test results with RIBA-II (i.e. single antigen positive), a preliminary report shows that when the single band is c-33 or c-22, HCV-RNA is detected in 88% and 48% of cases respectively. When the single band is c-100 or 5-1-1, HCV-RNA is not detected at all.[10] In a second study, all isolated c-22 reactivity results were felt to be false positive.[11]

However, disappointing results were obtained in recent quality control testing of 31 laboratories for PCR HCV-RNA testing. A coded panel of sera was submitted and only 16% of the laboratories earned a perfect score. Overall 11% of the negative samples were reported positive and 4% of the strongly-positive samples were reported negative.[12] Since PCR can amplify small amounts of material, contamination (false-positivity) is a great problem. Storage of specimens can decrease the PCR signal and variability of HCV genotypes may cause false negativity if the wrong primer is used. Further work on standardization of the PCR needs to be done.[12,13] PCR testing for HCV-RNA is not commercially available.

It is 4/00 Now.

Thus, there is no *gold standard* for hepatitis C testing at the current time.

There are two conditions in patients with liver disease where serological testing for HCV is confusing. These two conditions are autoimmune chronic active hepatitis and alcoholic liver disease.

Autoimmune hepatitis

Autoimmune hepatitis (AIH) is a multisystem disease characterized by inflammation of the liver that can lead to cirrhosis. Extrahepatic symptoms such as arthritis, pleurisy or colitis may accompany the liver disease. Persistent or recurrent jaundice commonly occurs in AIH. In contrast, jaundice seldom occurs in early chronic hepatitis C and extrahepatic involvement is rare (Table 9.2). Although AIH can affect all age and racial groups, it is most common in young Caucasian women. There is an 8:1 female to male ratio in AIH.[14]

Table 9.2 Features of autoimmune hepatitis. Used with permission. National Hepatitis Detection, Treatment and Prevention Program's Issues® in Hepatitis.

- 8:1 female to male ratio
- Eurocaucasian ancestry
- Extrahepatic involvement common (arthralgias, pleuritis, colitis)
- Jaundice common
- Hypergammaglobulinemia
- Presence of autoantibodies
- Corticosteroid responsive

In poorly understood ways, hepatitis C may occasionally be involved in the pathogenesis of AIH in some cases.[15, 16] Unfortunately there is weak correlation among the three available tests (EIA-2, RIBA-II, HCV-RNA) when AIH patients are tested for the presence of hepatitis C.[6, 15] The distinction between HCV and AIH is crucial since the treatments for each are immunologically different and improper treatment may worsen a patient with an incorrect diagnosis.[17–19] Patients with AIH who are positive for HCV on EIA testing, will often test negatively after prednisone treatment.[6, 17] Prednisone results in quick and dramatic improvement in aminotransferase values and symptoms of AIH.

In patients felt to have severe AIH, despite being positive for EIA-2 and HCV-RNA, prednisone did not help liver tests and in fact caused clinical deterioration of two patients.[20]

Alfa-interferon is clearly the treatment of choice for progressive liver disease due to hepatitis C (Chapter 9). However, when given to patients thought to have AIH, clinical deterioration occurs. If doubt exists as to the correct diagnosis, it is better to start with a course of prednisone rather than alfa-interferon. Prednisone is much less harmful to hepatitis C than alfa-interferon is to AIH. With either group of patients, a poor response or deterioration during therapy should cause reconsideration of the diagnosis and perhaps a switch to the alternative therapy.[17]

Alcoholic liver disease

Numerous reports show prevalence figures of 25 to 38% of patients with alcoholic liver disease to also test positive for hepatitis C.[21,22] Most reports have used the obsolete EIA-1 test and little data are available for EIA-2 among alcoholics. Fong et al. found 38% of patients with alcoholic liver disease to test positive with EIA-2.[22] RIBA-II or HCV-RNA testing will be positive 80 to 88% of the time when EIA-2 is positive.[22, 23] HCV-RNA is not found when the RIBA-II is negative.[23] Alcohol-related injury appears to be the predominant injury in RIBA-II positive patients.[23]

Hepatitis C positive alcoholic patients have a more severe histologic picture than HCV-negative alcoholics.[21] In the author's experience, the only patients with cirrhosis due to hepatitis C under age 50 are those who habitually (i.e., daily) imbibe alcohol.

Thus, confirmatory testing of positive EIA results in patients with alcoholic liver disease seems warranted. However, since alfa-interferon has not been used in patients with these two conditions co-existing, it is common sense to forbid alcohol for 6–12 months and repeat EIA-2 HCV testing upon follow-up.

Epidemiology and Transmission

Post-transfusion hepatitis

The clearest mode of infection by HCV is percutaneous transmission with contaminated blood. After introduction of markers for hepatitis A and B in 1974, the existence of post-transfusion non-A, non-B (PT-NANB) viral hepatitis became a diagnostic category. Prospective studies conducted in the 1970's and early 1980's estimated an infection rate of 5–18% depending on the amount of transfused product given.[24]

An attempt was made in the mid-1980's to lower the incidence of PT-NANB by screening blood products with "surrogate" markers. Surrogate markers are blood tests which seem to be associated with the presence of infectivity. Units of blood were tested for elevated concentrations of alanine aminotransferase (ALT) and for the presence of the IgG for hepatitis B core antibody (anti-HBc). Excluding units of blood positive for surrogate markers markedly reduced the incidence of PT-NANB (Table 9.3). Specific testing for HCV began in 1990 with EIA-1 and reduced the rate of PT-NANB hepatitis further to an incidence of 0.57% or a risk of 0.03% (about 1 in 3300) per unit of blood (Table 9.3).[24] EIA-2 testing further reduces the rate of infection by

Table 9.3 Rates of HCV seroconversion, according to the method used to screen donated blood. Reprinted, by permission of the *New England Journal of Medicine*, vol. 327; page 371, 1992.

Type of Screening	Sero-Conversion	Patients at Risk	Units Transfused	Sero-Conversion Rate	
				Per patient	Per unit
				percent	
Routine only	35	912	7810	3.84	0.45
Routine plus surrogate markers	15	976	8015	1.54	0.19
Routine plus surrogate markers and anti-HCV	3	522	9916	0.57	0.03

20–50%.[5] The current risk of PT-NANB (and EIA-2 negative) hepatitis appears to range from 0.05% (1 in 2000) to 0.017% (1 in 6000) per unit of blood transfusion.[25]

The explanation for continued existence of post-transfusion hepatitis may be twofold. First, there are donors who test negative for all sensitive assays except by the PCR HCV-RNA test.[26] Secondly, another non-A, non-B percutaneously transmitted virus may exist. This virus has been long suspected but its existence is controversial. Rather than refer to this suspected agent as non-A, non-B, non-C, non-E virus, it is easier to use the proposed designation of hepatitis G.[27]

Hemophilia

All hemophiliacs who received clotting factor concentrates prior to the late 1980's have been infected with HCV. Seroprevalence rates with confirmatory assays range from 91 to 99%.[28, 29] It is likely that those few patients who are seronegative have had the virus and subsequently cleared it.[30] HCV is found more frequently in hemophiliacs co-infected with HIV.[29,31]

Starting about 1988, heat and other means of viral inactivation have nearly eliminated the risk of any type of viral transmission from blood derived clotting factors.[29,31]

Co-infected hemophiliac patients with HCV and HIV appear to have more rapidly progressive disease and higher levels of viremia.[32] The subject of coinfection is reviewed in detail in Chapter 11.

Ultimately, as many as 5–10% of patients with hemophilia and HCV alone die of chronic liver disease.[33]

Needle exposure

Intravenous drug abuse.
Intravenous drug abuse (IVDA) is another risk group with almost universal HCV infection. Studies with confirmatory testing show seroprevalence figures of 64 to 85%. HIV infection does not appear to increase HCV prevalence in IVDA.[34,35] HCV infection spreads rapidly in this population as evidenced by a 70% prevalence rate in those reporting IVDA for less than one year.[34]

In the author's practice, IVDA is the most common cause of HCV infection and accounts for more than half of those referred for HCV evaluation. IVDA also accounts for the most common cause of "occult" HCV infection. The author has had many patients referred who allegedly have no risk factor for acquisition of HCV. If they are in the 30 to 45 year old age group, gentle questioning often reveals a brief period of IV drug experimentation. Patients who have previously denied "intravenous drug abuse" will often admit to "trying IV drugs once" when they were younger. Many of these patients who admit to brief intravenous drug use are now upstanding citizens in the community and for whom the phrase "intravenous drug abuse" connotes all sorts of wild pictures and behaviors.

Needlestick accident.
Accidental exposure from a needle contaminated by blood from a known hepatitis C carrier occurs in health care workers. Kiyosawa, et al., followed 110 medical workers exposed to an anti-HCV positive (EIA-1) needlestick.[36] Four patients (4%) developed hepatitis and three seroconverted with anti-HCV. Jaundice developed in three workers after 33 to 46 days and the ALT level exceeded 10× normal. One recipient became a chronic carrier.

Mitsui et al. followed 68 health care workers similarly exposed to an HCV contaminated needlestick.[37] Testing was performed with the more sensitive HCV-RNA PCR assay. Seven personnel (10%) became infected. The hepatitis among these seven was subclinical and self-limited except for one recipient who had persistent ALT elevations and anti-HCV on long-term follow-up.

Needlestick inoculation may inject 10^5–10^6 fewer HCV virions than a transfusion of a unit of HCV-positive blood; thus, the transmission rate should be much lower than the 80% occurrence rate among recipients of a known anti-HCV positive unit of blood.[36, 37]

Tattooing is a similar risk factor for acquiring HCV infection. In one study with the RIBA-II assay, 12.6% of tattooed subjects were anti-HCV positive versus 2.4% of controls. Positive results for HCV correlated with an increasing number of tattoos and whether or not the injections were done by a professional.[38]

Sexual transmission

>> *The following section comments on what may be the most contro-versial area in viral hepatitis, namely the vexing problem of possi-ble sexual transmission of HCV. The general reader may not wish to read this detailed evaluation which concludes that sexual trans-mission occurs rarely or not at all. The Centers for Disease Control has advised that monogamous couples, where one partner is in-fected with HCV, need not use condoms or change sexual habits.*

Early data about the possible sexual transmission of non-A, non-B/type C hepatitis gave conflicting information. The epidemiology of non-A, non-B (NANB) hepatitis suggested a weak association between the number of heterosexual contacts and the prevalence of NANB. However, first generation enzyme immunoassay hepatitis C (HCV) testing of the male homosexual community did not show an increased prevalence of HCV over the general population.

The Centers for Disease Control (CDC) 1989 report suggested an increased prevalence of NANB hepatitis in heterosexual patients with multiple sexual partners.[39] This broad-based epidemiological study did not have sexual transmission as the principal focus. Cases were attributed to intravenous drug abuse (IVDA) or blood transfusion only if these events occurred within six months of the epidemiological interview. HCV testing had not yet become available.

A follow-up CDC study in 1990 looked at the same subjects pre-viously reported and tested them with EIA-1.[40] Only two-thirds of patients originally thought to have NANB hepatitis tested positive for HCV.[40]

Three methodological criticisms, in retrospect, invalidate these two related articles. First, limiting assignment of IVDA to those reporting the behavior in the prior six months overestimates the pool of "un-known source." A substantial proportion of all HCV cases are caused by IVDA and almost all members of this risk group have been infected with HCV.[34,41] Secondly, one-third of cases in the 1989 report are, in reality, non-A, non-B, non-C cases. Thirdly, EIA 1.0 anti-HCV testing may have as high as 70% false positivity in a low risk population (i.e., no prior blood transfusions or IVDA).[42] In retrospect, since the two prior articles have so many methodological problems, they should be disregarded. Unfortunately, the author encounters many who still cite them for support of sexual transmission.

The CDC has since performed a focused study of sexual transmission, with EIA 1.0 testing, and concluded sexual activity was not associated with transmission of HCV. Furthermore, in the study population of those having multiple sexual partners, HCV positivity was largely associated with IVDA.[43]

The marked disparity between the prevalence of hepatitis B and C in the homosexual population has provided evidence for a long time that hepatitis C is either rarely sexually transmitted or not at all. In contrast to hepatitis C, hepatitis B is clearly sexually transmitted among homosexuals with a sero-prevalence rate of 50–95%. A recent report of 735 homosexual men from San Francisco showed 34 (4.6%) to test positive for HCV by RIBA-II.[44] However, 27 had a history of intravenous drug abuse or prior blood transfusions, leaving only seven (0.95%) without obvious risk factors for HCV acquisition. The prevalence rate of 0.95% is within the general population range of 0.3% to 1.7%.[42,45] The low seroprevalence of HCV is remarkable since bleeding can occur during rectal intercourse and many homosexuals report a large number of sexual partners.[44,46]

Returning to heterosexual couples, in a well done California study of a population with multiple risk factors, positivity for HCV by RIBA-II was *not* associated with any type of sexual practice (including intercourse during menstruation); however, positivity was again strongly related to IVDA.[35]

In reviewing all of the articles on the prevalence of HCV in spouses that use supplemental testing, a clear dichotomy of results seems to occur between Western and Oriental reports (Tables 9.4 and 9.5).

When spouses with other risk factors are subtracted from Western studies, the seroprevalence rate is 0.82% (4/489) [95% confidence interval 0.41% to 1.23%] a figure which is not different from the general population prevalence of 0.3 to 1.7%.

Some of the studies, which include the length of sexual exposure, report an extremely long marriage for cohorts. Esteban et al. reported a mean contact time of 23 years for couples in his study.[50] Given an average frequency of sexual intercourse, two to three times per week reported by many researchers in marriage, the risk translates to greater

Table 9.4 Western studies of HCV seroprevalence among heterosexual partners. Only studies which use supplementary testing are included.

Author	HCV Methodology	# Positive/Total	# Spouses with other risk factors	# Positive (no other risk factors)	Risk Factors
Luba[47]	RNA	0/20	–	0/20	
Gordon[48]	RIBA-II/RNA	2/42	2	0/40	IVDA, razor sharing
Brettler[49]	RIBA-II	3/104	3	0/101	IVDA, nurse, HIV+
Esteban[50]	RIBA-II	2/86	2	0/84	Blood transfusion, prior hepatitis
Deny[51]	RIBA-II	0/30	–	0/30	
Kolho[52]	RIBA-II	0/30	–	0/30	
Bresters[53]	RIBA-II/RNA	0/50	–	0/50	
Buscarini[45]	RIBA-II	5/34	1	4/33	Syringe use
Hallam[54]	RNA	3/104	3	0/101	IVDA, blood transfusion
TOTALS %		15/500 3%		4/489 0.82%	

than 160,000 exposures per couple without HCV transmission occurring. Bresters study from the Netherlands shows all 50 partners negative for RIBA-II and HCV-RNA after a calculated 713 person-years of unprotected sexual intercourse.[53] The large number of sexual contacts in the latter two studies would seem to make the possibility of a low level risk of transmission quite unlikely.

On the other hand, the seroprevalence rates of Oriental spouses (Table 9.5) are much greater. With and without other risk factors being subtracted, the prevalence rates are 9.5 and 10.7%, respectively.

Higher prevalence rates in the Orient do not prove causality of sexual transmission. Three confounding problems exist when trying to interpret Oriental spousal data. First, the prevalence of HCV in the population is much higher and ranges from 0.9%–32.4%, depending on the age of blood donors.[57, 61, 61A] Secondly, five of the six Oriental studies utilized only HCV-RNA and not RIBA-II and the HCV-RNA assay can easily have false positive results which can be controlled for

Table 9.5 Oriental studies of HCV seroprevalence among heterosexual partners. Only studies which use supplementary testing are included.

Author	HCVSupplemental Methodology	# Positive/Total	# Spouses with Other Risk Factors	# Positive (No Other Risk Factors)/total	Risk Factors
Wang[55]	RNA	0/11	–	0/11	
Terado[56]	RNA	0/3	–	0/3	
Oshita[57]	RIBA-II/RNA	13/75	–	13/75	
Kao[58]	RNA	7/38	?	7/38	
Alcahane[59]	RNA	14/176	?	14/176	IVDA not mentioned
Mizokami[60]	RNA	6/70	5	1/65	Divergence times differ (see text)
TOTALS		40/373		35/368	
%		10.72%		9.5%	

by the highly specific RIBA-II test. In contrast, seven of nine western studies utilized RIBA-II testing.

The third confounding factor is that husband and wife may have been infected through common external sources such as razor sharing or acupuncture. 40–50% of Japanese HCV carriers report a history of acupuncture or other percutaneous folk remedies.[61, 61A] 17% of ethnic Chinese men report a history of acupuncture.[62] Multiple epidemics of acupuncture associated hepatitis B have been reported[62] and it is logical that HCV could be spread in this manner. 11/283 HCV carriers in Japan report tattooing or intravenous drug abuse (IVDA).[61] A study from Taiwan shows a strong association between tattooing and acquisition of HCV.[38] Oriental reports are often silent about IVDA or report an extremely low percentage.[58,59] It is not certain whether IVDA is truly rare in the Orient or whether it is underreported since IVDA is the most common risk factor in HCV carriers reported in Western studies of HCV carriers.

Further support for the concept that increased prevalence of HCV among Oriental spouses represents something other than sexual transmission comes from a recent Japanese abstract which reported six of 70

Table 9.6 PCR HCV-RNA testing of body fluids from chronic HCV carriers. Data derived from references 56, 64, 65.

National Institues of Health	
Saliva, semen—14 males	None detected
Stanford	
Saliva, urine, semen, stool, vaginal secretions, breast milk—15 carriers	None detected
Japan	
Urine, semen—6 males	None detected

spouses to be positive by EIA 2.0 and HCV-RNA.[30] HCV mutates at a regular rate. This group used the mutation rate to construct a phylogenetic tree to estimate the divergence time between husband and wife's strains. There was only one couple whose divergence time was shorter than their marriage period. The other five couples had longer divergence times suggesting non-marital exposure.[60]

Obtaining a history of risk factors for HCV is fraught with obtaining false answers. This history taking problem is obviated in an experimental population of 85 chimpanzees in Japan where 13 animals were infected with HCV and followed for ten years. No sexual or mother to infant transmission occurred despite 39 chimpanzees being born during the observation time period.[63]

In an effort to clarify a possible (or absent) mechanism of sexual transmission, investigators at the National Institutes of Health (NIH) tested the saliva and semen of 14 male chronic carriers for HCV-RNA (Table 9.6). No evidence of HCV in these secretions was discovered by this sensitive assay. Blood from each carrier was then added to every sample of saliva and semen and tested again. All samples subsequently tested positive for RNA; and this serves to exclude an inhibiting substance or other reason for false negativity.[63]

At Stanford University Medical Center, 15 chronic carriers had saliva, urine, semen, stool, vaginal secretions and breast milk examined for HCV-RNA and all body secretions were negative. Again, as in the NIH study, added blood caused samples to become positive for HCV-RNA.[65]

A third study from Japan also reported no evidence of HCV-RNA in urine or semen of six infected patients.[56] A fourth study showed 7 of 14 carriers to test HCV-RNA positive in saliva. However, 13 of the 14 salivary samples were reactive for hemocult testing suggesting blood contamination of the salivary samples.[55] One important methodological difference in the latter study from the NIH and Stanford series is that investigators took whole saliva rather than clarified saliva. Clarification involves removing cells from the saliva before extracting the RNA. Whether clarification has a detrimental effect on testing of saliva is unknown.[41] There are no food-associated epidemics of hepatitis C. Oral transmission of HCV by saliva is felt to be highly unlikely.[41]

The negative results of testing for HCV-RNA in body fluids are remarkable to this author since contamination (or false positivity) remains a problem rather than sensitivity (i.e., false negativity) with the PCR assay.

Given the low prevalence of HCV in homosexuals and western heterosexuals, the absence of transmission in chimpanzee colonies and the undetectability of HCV in sexual body secretions, it can be concluded that sexual transmission occurs extremely rarely or not at all.

The increased prevalence seen in oriental spouses is probably due to an increased percutaneous exposure outside of marriage in the form of acupuncture or other modalities.

Teaching should reflect the concept of non-transmission. As an analogy, it is taught that hepatitis A is not transmitted by blood transfusions; yet, a few cases are reported.[66] The viremic phase of hepatitis A is brief and transmission through a unit of blood requires having an asymptomatic infected person donate blood during this short period of viremia.

Sexual transmission for hepatitis C (if it occurs at all) appears to be on the same order of magnitude as transmitting hepatitis A with blood transfusion. Therefore, it is reasonable to teach that transmission in either case does not occur.

Some writers still consider sexual transmission as uncommon but significant:

> Patients with long-standing monogamous relationships ...should be made aware of the inconclusive nature of the data on HCV sexual transmission...[and] reassurance should be conveyed. Thereafter, the decision to alter sexual practices can be deferred to patients and their partners.[67]

It should be noted that the above recommendation, published in August, 1993 by a caucus group, cited the 1990 CDC investigation. The 1990 study, while the best available at the time, has been superseded by better studies with more sensitive and specific serology.

The author encounters extreme anxiety from couples over the sexual transmission issue. Patients need comfort and reassurance with a straightforward yes or no answer. Most patients cannot understand a discussion of low probability. Words like "maybe," "possible," "rarely," do little to calm the extreme agitation many couples have and may cause destruction of interpersonal relationships.

The CDC agrees that data for sexual transmission of hepatitis C is meager and officially recommends that precautions (i.e., condoms) or changes in sexual habits are unnecessary among monogamous couples where one partner is chronically infected with HCV.[68] The recent evidence against sexual transmission reviewed here clearly supports continuing the current CDC advisory. Enough scientific information is now available to support the contention that sexual transmission of HCV occurs extremely rarely, or more likely, not at all.

Household contacts.
An early study by the NIH, with EIA-1 testing, of 62 household and sexual contacts reported no contacts to be HCV positive.[69]

Two other EIA-1 studies found 6% of 34 family members and 8% of 88 family members anti-HCV positive.[68] However, when second generation RIBA-II or HCV-RNA testing has been done, no family members (106 in France, 27 in U.S.) without other risk factors have been positive for HCV.[47, 51] Thus, intrafamilial transmission appears very low or non-existent. It is clear that HCV is not transmitted through the fecal-oral route since there are no reports of food associated epidemics as in case of hepatitis A. There is no evidence that sneezing, coughing or casual contact transmits HCV.[68]

However, household items of a carrier that can become contaminated with blood (e.g., razors, toothbrushes) should not be shared. Also, cuts or skin lesions should be covered to prevent blood contact.[68]

Organ donation.
Virtually all HCV negative recipients of solid organs (e.g., heart, kidney, liver) from HCV positive donors become infected with hepatitis C.[70] Whether the resulting liver disease is significant, or worth the 2–8% wastage of organs if HCV donors are excluded, is controversial.[71]

The CDC recommends that hepatitis C carriers not donate blood, body organs, other tissue, or semen.[68]

Maternal infant transmission.
In a U.S. study of 24 infants born to HCV infected mothers, none of the babies followed for three to six months after delivery had evidence for HCV infection as tested by HCV-RNA.[72] A Swedish study followed 21

newborns and only one infant became persistently positive for HCV-RNA and developed biochemical hepatitis.[73]

Transmission may be higher if the mother is co-infected with the HIV virus. A French study of eight mothers, infected with both viruses, showed three infants with HCV-RNA present at birth; only one of which developed chronic aminotransferase elevations and persistent HCV-RNA.[74] In an earlier study of 43 infants from HCV positive mothers (tested by first generation RIBA) the only infants with evidence of chronic HCV infection were also infected with HIV virus. Four infants had both HCV and HIV from a total of nine HIV infected infants.[75]

In the latest study from Japan, the risk or transmission appeared to be related to viral replication levels in the mother.[13,76] Six percent of EIA-2 positive mother (3 of 53) transmitted HCV to their offspring. However, only 31 of 53 mothers had detectable HCV-RNA and 11% of these mothers transmitted HCV compared to none of the HCV-RNA negative mothers. Further, transmission only occurred if the titer of HCV-RNA was greater than 10^6 per ml.[76]

Thus, outside of coinfection with HIV, maternal-infant transmission appears low. However, concern has been expressed over the sensitivity and specificity of HCV assays in neonates and the possibility that late seroconversion (i.e., >15 months) may occur.[77]

Community-acquired HCV.

Sporadic occurrence of HCV is defined as a patient with HCV and no known risk factors. Further, the patient denies IVDA, prior blood transfusions and has no tattoos.

Early studies suggested the sporadic occurrence may be as high as 40% but the author's experience and others[41] shows fewer than 5% of HCV cases lack any of the major percutaneous risk factors. The earlier caveat, about denial of IVDA in those born after 1945, needs to be taken seriously. Subjects with a remote history of IVDA are reluctant to admit such behavior to an interviewer. In addition, patients may be uninformed as to whether blood products were received during prior surgical procedures.

Fecal-oral transmission and sexual activity do not appear to account for sporadic occurrence. Maternal-infant transmission is quite low but may account for an occasional sporadic case.

It is likely, therefore, that genuine sporadic acquisition does not occur. Community-acquired HCV is likely due to either denial or ignorance about known risk actors such as IVDA, blood products or inapparent percutaneous exposure.

Summary of Diagnosis and Transmission of Hepatitis C

1. Hepatitis C is diagnosed with the EIA-2 HCV antibody. If the patient has a known risk factor such as prior blood transfusions or intravenous drug use and abnormal serum aminotransferases, no supplemental testing is needed.
2. RIBA-II testing increases the specificity of EIA-2 results but not sensitivity. RIBA-II testing is indicated in:
   - Patient with no known risk factors
   - Normal ALT levels
   - Alcoholic liver disease
3. If autoimmune chronic active hepatitis is suspected, all current tests for HCV (EIA-2, RIBA-II, HCV-RNA) may give conflicting or misleading results. Clinical judgement is required and a trial of corticosteroids should be considered first rather than alfa-interferon.
4. The role of sexual transmission is not yet completely evaluated. Data thus far indicate either that transmission occurs extremely rarely or not at all. Changes among sexual practices of monogamous couples are not recommended. Similarly, household transmission appears rare. Household members of a chronic HCV carrier should avoid sharing blood contaminated items such as razors and tooth brushes. Open wounds of a carrier should be adequately covered.
5. Maternal-infant transmission appears to happen infrequently and the presence of HCV should not discourage pregnancy or vaginal delivery (see Chapter 11).

References

1. Alter HJ, Purcell RH, Feinstone SM, et al. Non-A, non-B hepatitis: its relationship to cytomegalovirus, to chronic hepatitis, and to direct and indirect test methods. In: Szmuness W, Alter HJ, Maynard JE, eds. *Viral Hepatitis: 1981 Symposium:* Franklin Institute Press, 1982:279–294.
2. Editorial. Will the real hepatitis C stand up? *Lancet* 1989; 2:307-8.
3. Choo QL, Kuo G, Weiner AJ, et al. Isolation of a cDNA clone derived from a blood-borne non-A, non-B viral hepatitis genome. *Science* 1989; 244:359–361.
4. Kuo G, Choo QL, Alter HJ, et al. An assay for circulating antibodies to a major etiologic virus of human non-A, non-B hepatitis. *Science* 1989; 244:362–364.

5. Alter HJ. New kit on the block: evaluation of second-generation assays for detection of antibody to the hepatitis C virus. *Hepatology* 1992; 15:350–353.

6. McHutchison JG, Person JL, Govindarajan S, et al. Improved detection of hepatitis C virus antibodies in high-risk populations. *Hepatology* 1992; 15:1–25.

7. Van der poel CL, Cuypers HM, Reesink HW, et al. Confirmation of hepatitis C virus infection by new four-antigen recombinant immuoblot assay. *Lancet* 1991; 337:317–319.

8. Serfaty L, Giral P, Elghouzzi ME, et al. Risk factors for hepatitis C virus infection in hepatitis C antibody ELISA-positive blood donors according to RIBA-2 status: a case control survey. *Hepatology* 1993; 17:183–187.

9. Package Insert. ORTHO® HCV 2.0 Elisa Test System. Ortho Diagnostic Systems, Inc. Raritan, NJ.

10. Li X, Reddy R, Jeffers L, et al. Evaluation of indeterminate hepatitis C RIBA-II sera by RT-PCR. *Hepatology* 1992; 16:73A (abstract).

11. Tobler LH, Busch MP, Wilber J, et al. Evaluation of indeterminate c22-3 reactivity in volunteer blood donors. *Transfusion* 1994; 34: 130–134.

12. Zaaijer HL, Cuypers HM, Reesink HW, et al. Reliability of polymerase chain reaction for detection of hepatitis C virus. *Lancet* 1993; 341:722–724.

13. Alter MJ. Transmission of hepatitis C virus-route, dose, and titer. *N Engl J Med* 1994; 330:784–785.

14. What disease is this? *Issues in Hepatitis Winter 1992*; 2:1-4. (Published by Advanced Therapeutic Communications, Secaucus, NJ 07094)

15. Nishiguchi S, Kuroki T, Ueda T, et al. Detection of hepatitis C virus antibody in the absence of viral RNA in patients with autoimmune hepatitis. *Ann Int Med* 1992; 116:21–25.

16. Editorial. HCV and autoimmune liver disease. *Lancet* 1990; 336:1414–1415.

17. Martin P. Hepatitis C: from laboratory to bedside. *Mayo Clin Proc* 1990; 65:1372–1376.

18. Black M. Alpha-interferon treatment of chronic hepatitis C: need for accurate diagnosis in selecting patients. Ann Int Med 1992; 116:86–88.

19. Papo T, Marcellin P, Bernuau J, et al. Authoimmune chronic hepatitis exacerbated by alpha-interferon. *Ann Int Med* 1992; 116:51–53.

20. Magrin S, Craxi A, Fabiano C, et al. HCV-RNA in severe "autoimmune" chronic active hepatitis. *Hepatology* 1992; 16:211 (abstract).

21. Caldwell SH, Jeffers LJ, Ditomaso A, et al. Antibody to hepatitis C is common among patients with alcoholic liver disease with and without risk factors. *Am J Gastroenterology* 1991; 86:1219–1223.

22. Fong TL, Karel GC, Conrad A, et al. Clinical significance of concomitant hepatitis C infection in patients with alcoholic liver disease. *Hepatology* 1994; 19:554–557.

23. Nalpas B, Thiers V, Pol S, et al. Hepatitis C viremia and anti-HCV antibodies in alcoholics. *J Hepatology* 1992; 14:381–384.

24. Donahue JG, Munoz AM, Ness PM, et al. The declining risk of post-transfusion hepatitis C virus infection. *N Engl J Med* 1992; 327:369–373.

25. Kleinman S, Busch M, Holland P, et al. Post transfusion hepatitis C virus infection. *N Engl J Med* 1992; 327:1601–1602.

26. Sugitani M, Inchauspe G, Shindo M, et al. Sensitivity of serological assays to identify blood donors with hepatitis C viremia. *Lancet* 1992; 339:1018–1019.

27. Editorial. The A to F of viral hepatitis. *Lancet* 1990; 336:1158–1160.

28. Watson HG, Ludlam CA, Rebus S, et al. Use of several second generation assays to determine the true prevalence of hepatitis C virus infection in haemophiliacs treated with non-virus inactivated factor VIII and IX concentrates. *Br J Haematol* 1992; 80:514—518.

29. Allain JP, Dailey SH, Laurion Y, et al. Evidence for persistent hepatitis C virus infection in hemophiliacs. *J Clin Invest* 1991; 88:1672—1679.

30. Simmonds P, Zhang LQ, Watson HG, et al. Hepatitis C quantification and sequencing in blood products, haemophilics and drug users. *Lancet* 1990; 336:1469–1472.

31. Julius C, Westphal RG. The safety of blood components and derivatives. *Hemat Oncol Clinics of North America* 1992; 6:1057–1077.

32. Watson HG, Zhang LQ, Simmonds P, et al. Hepatitis C virus load increases with time after HIV infection. *Int Conf Aids* 1992; 8:B195 (abstract #PoB 3629).

33. Alter HJ. Chronic consequences of non-A, non-B hepatitis. In: Seeff LB, Lewis JH, eds. *Current Perspectives in Hepatology*. New York:: Plenum, 1989:83–97.

34. Donahue JG, Nelson KE, Munoz A, et al. Antibody to hepatitis C virus among cardiac surgery patients, homosexual men, and intravenous drug users in Baltimore, Maryland. *Am J Epidemiology*: 1991; 134:1206–1211.

35. Osmond DH, Padian NS, Sheppard HW, et al. Risk factors for hepatitis C virus seropositivity in heterosexual couples. *JAMA* 1993; 269:361–365.

36. Kiyosawa K, Sodeyama T, Tanaka E, et al. Hepatitis C in hospital employees with Needlestick injuries. *Ann Intern Med* 1991; 115:367–369.
37. Mitsui T, Iwano K, Maksuka K, et al. Hepatitis C virus infection in medical personnel after needlestick accident. *Hepatology* 1992; 16:1109–1114.
38. Ko YC, Ho MS, Chiang TA, et al. Tattooing as a risk of hepatitis C virus infection. *J Med Virology* 1992; 38:288–291.
39. Alter MJ, Coleman PJ, Alexander WJ, et al. Importance of heterosexual activity in the transmission of hepatitis B and non-A, non-B hepatitis. *JAMA* 1989; 262:1201–1205.
40. Alter MJ, Hadler SC, Judson FN, et al. Risk factors for acute non-A, non-B hepatitis in the United States and association with hepatits C virus infection. *JAMA* 1990; 264:2231–2235.
41. Hollinger FB, Lin HJ. Community-acquired hepatitis C virus infection. *Gastroenterology* 1992; 102:1426–1429.
42. Alter HJ. Descartes before the horse: I clone, therefore I am: the hepatitis C virus in current perspective. *Ann Intern Med* 1991; 115:644–649.
43. Weinstock HS, Bolan G, Reingold AC, et al. Hepatitis C virus infection among patients attending a clinic for sexually transmitted diseases. *JAMA* 1993; 269:392–394.
44. Osmond DH, Charlesbois E, Sheppard HW, et al. Comparison of risk factors for hepatitis C and hepatitis B infection in homosexual men. *J Infect Dis* 1993; 167:66–71.
45. Buscarini E, Tanzi E, Zanetti AR, et al. High prevalence of antibodies to hepatitis C virus among family members of patients with anti-HCV positive chronic liver disease. *Scand J Gastroenterology* 1993; 28:343–346.
46. Reiner NE, Judson FN, Bond WW, et al. Asymptomatic rectal mucosal lesions and hepatitis B surface antigen at sites of sexual contact in homosexual men with persistent hepatitis B infection. *Ann Intern Med* 1982; 96:170–173.
47. Luba D, Hsu H, Martin MC, et al. Failure of transmission of hepatitis C through household or sexual contact. *Hepatology* 1992; 14:77A.
48. Gordon SC, Patel AH, Kulesza GW, et al. Lack of evidence for the heterosexual transmission of hepatitis C. *Am J Gast* 1992; 87:1849–1851.
49. Brettler DB, Mannucci PM, Gringeri A, et al. The low risk of hepatitis C virus transmission among sexual partners of hepatitis

C infected hemophiliac males: an international multicenter study. *Blood* 1992; 80:540–543.

50. Esteban JI, Lopez-Talavera JC, Genesca J, et al. High rate of infectivity and liver disease in blood donors with antibodies to hepatitis C virus. *Ann Intern Med* 1991; 115:443–449.

51. Deny P, Roulot D, Asselot C, et al. Low rate of hepatitis C virus (HCV) transmission within the family. *J Hepat* 1992; 14:409–410.

52. Kolho E, Naukkarinen R, Ebeling F, et al. Transmission of hepatitis C virus to sexual partners of seropositive patients with bleeding disorders: a rare event. *Scan J Inf Dis* 1991; 23:667–670.

53. Bresters D, Mauser-Bunschoten EP, Reesink HW, et al. Sexual transmission of hepatitis C virus. *Lancet* 1993; 342:210–211.

54. Hallam NF, Fletcher ML, Read SJ, et al. Low risk of sexual transmission of hepatitis C virus. *J Med Virology* 1993; 40:251–253.

55. Wang JT, Wang TH, Sheu JC, et al. Hepatitis C virus RNA in saliva with post-transfusion hepatitis and low efficiency of transmission among spouses. *J Med Virology* 1992; 36:28–31.

56. Terada S, Kawanishi K, Katayama K. Minimal hepatitis C infectivity in semen. *Ann Intern Med* 1992; 117:171.

57. Oshita M, Hayashi N, Kasahara A, et al. Prevalence of hepatitis C virus in family members of patients with hepatitis C. *J Med Virology* 1993; 41:251–255.

58. Kao JH, Chen PJ, Yang PM, et al. Intrafamilial transmission of hepatitis C virus: the important role of infections between spouses. *J Infect Dis* 1992; 166:900–903.

59. Akahane Y, Aikawa T, Sugai Y, Tsuda F, Okamoto H, Mishiro S. Transmission of HCV between spouses. *Lancet* 1992; 339:1059–1060.

60. Mizokami M, Ohno T, Ina Y, et al. Sexual transmission of hepatitis C virus. *Hepatology* 1993; 18:244 (abstract).

61A.Kiyosawa K, Tanaka E, Sodeyama T, et al. Transmission of hepatitis C in an isolated area in Japan: community-acquired infection. *Gastroenterology* 1994; 106:1596-1602.

61. Shimoyama R, Sekiguchi S, Suga M, et al. The epidemiology and infection route of asymptomatic HCV carriers detected through blood donations. *Gastroenterologica Japonica* 1993; 28 (suppl. 5):1-5.

62. Phoon WO, Fong NP, Lee J. History of blood transfusion, tattooing, acupuncture and risk of hepatitis B surface antigenaemia among Chinese men in Singapore. *Am J Pub Health* 1988; 78:958–960.

63. Suzuki E, Kaneko S, Udono T, et al. Absence of nonpercutaneous transmission of hepatitis C virus in a colony of chimpanzees. *J Med Virology* 1993; 39:286–291.

64. Fried MW, Shindo M, Fong TL, et al. Absence of hepatitis C viral RNA from saliva and semen of patients with chronic hepatitis C. *Gastroenterology* 1992; 102:1306–1308.

65. Hsu H, Wright TL, Luba D, et al. Is hepatitis C virus in human secretions? . *Gastroenterology* 1991; 100:754 (abstract).

66. Hollinger FB, Khan NC, Oefinger PE, et al. Post-transfusion hepatitis type A. *JAMA* 1983; 250:2313–2317.

67. Sexual transmission of hepatitis C: What to tell patients. *Issues in Hepatitis* 1993; 3:2-3. (Available from Advanced Therapeutics Communications, 400 Plaza Drive, Secaucus, NJ 07094)

68. Centers for Disease Control. Public Health Service inter-agency guidelines for screening donors of blood, plasma, organs, tissues, and semen for evidence of hepatitis B and C. *MMWR* 1991; 40:RR-4.

69. Everhart JE, Di Bisceglie AM, Murry LM, et al. Risk for non-A, non-B (Type C) hepatitis through sexual or household contact with chronic carriers. *Ann Intern Med* 1990; 112:544–545.

70. Pereira BJ, Milford EL, Kirkman RL, et al. Prevalence of hepatitis C virus RNA in organ donors positive for hepatitis C antibody and in the recipients of their organs. *N Engl J Med* 1992; 327:910–915.

71. Morales JM, Andres A, Campistol JM, et al. Hepatitis C virus and organ transplantation. *N Engl J Med* 1993; 328:511–515.

72. Reinus JF, Leikin EL, Alter HJ, et al. Failure to detect vertical transmission of hepatitis C virus. *Ann Intern Med* 1992; 117:881–886.

73. Wejstal R, Widell A, Mansson AS, et al. Mother-to-infant transmission of hepatitis C virus. *Ann Intern Med* 1992; 117:887–890.

74. Novati R, Thiers V, Monforte AA, et al. Mother-to-child transmission of hepatitis C virus detected by nested polymerase chain reaction. *J Infect Dis* 1992; 165:720–723.

75. Weintrub PS, Veereman-Wauters G, Cowan MJ, et al. Hepatitis C virus infection in infants whose mothers took street drugs intravenously. *J Peds* 1991; 119:869–874.

76. Ohto H, Terazawa S, Sasaki N, et al. Transmission of hepatitis C virus from mothers to infants. *N Engl J Med* 1994; 330:744–750.

77. Koff RS. The low efficiency of maternal-neonatal transmission of hepatitis C virus: how certain are we? *Ann Intern Med* 1992; 117:967–968.

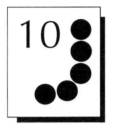

Clinical Features of Hepatitis C

Clinical Features
Pathology
Natural History
Complications
Clinical Evaluation

Clinical Features

Few studies report symptoms associated with the onset of hepatitis C. Most studies date from the time period before the availability of serology for HCV. Before the advent of specific testing, the disease was known as non-A, non-B (NANB) hepatitis. Post-transfusion studies, where the virus was identified as post-transfusion NANB (PT-NANB), provide the clearest understanding of the NANB virus. Retrospective testing has shown 90% of PT-NANB cases to be due to hepatitis C. Thus, while the NANB literature may not contain a single virus, the reported clinical picture is valid until studies using hepatitis C serology are performed.

Most patients with acute hepatitis C do not have signs or symptoms of the disease. In a consecutive study of 50 HCV patients discovered by blood donor screening, only 12% had a past history of symptomatic hepatitis;[1] furthermore, some of these 12% may be recounting an acute hepatitis A event (the most common cause of a past "jaundice" event).

Thus, most hepatitis C infections are anicteric. PT-NANB occurs after a mean incubation period of 7.8 weeks. The range is 2–26 weeks but 80–90% of cases occur within 5–12 weeks after transfusion.[2]

25% of acute PT-NANB cases develop jaundice.[2, 3] This is a similar proportion to hepatitis B; however, the bilirubin levels in PT-NANB tend to be much lower.[3,4] One-third of PT-NANB patients are quite symptomatic with ALT levels > 800 IU.[3] The remaining PT-NANB patients have mild disease detected only with serial aminotransferase levels.[2]

Chronic carriers of hepatitis C are often asymptomatic and discovered incidentally. The most common symptom in a clinical study of 102 consecutively referred patients to a liver unit was fatigue in 35%.[5] the mean serum aminotransferase levels were not different in those presenting with fatigue compared to those diagnosed incidentally. Again, only 18% of patients gave a past history of hepatitis or jaundice.[5]

Pathology

An excellent multicenter effort comparing 317 HCV biopsy specimens to 299 HBV samples gave four histological features that are clearly associated with the presence of HCV. These four features are *lymphoid aggregates/follicles* (Figure 10.1), *large droplet fat* (Figure 10.2) *bile duct damage* and *Mallory body-like material*.[6] (Illustrations of bile duct damage and Mallory body-like material can be found in Reference 6.)

Lymphoid structures such as follicles or aggregates are often present in autoimmune diseases. These structures are formed early in the acute stage of hepatitis C. However, overlapping of all four features occurs in acute and chronic HCV disease, making the distinction of acute from chronic disease difficult on purely pathological grounds.

Bile duct damage is found in about a third of biopsies for hepatitis C.[6,7] Bile duct damage occurs in many diseases such as primary biliary cirrhosis, drug toxicity and liver transplant rejection. Duct damage in hepatitis C, in contrast to other settings, does not appear to progress to duct destruction.[6] Despite the bile duct damage elevation of serum alkaline phosphatase does not occur in chronic hepatitis C.[8]

Fatty change and Mallory body-like material within hepatocytes fall into a category of "cytopathic" changes. These may occur as a result of direct cytotoxic affect of HCV on the hepatocyte.[6]

Scheuer and Sherlock comment that the presence of lymphoid aggregates together with an overall diagnosis of mild chronic active hepatitis (CAH) or chronic persistent hepatitis (CPH), fatty change

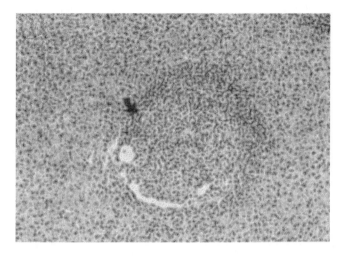

Figure 10.1 Lymphoid follicle with germinal center within portal tract in chronic hepatitis C. Note proximity of the follicle to the bile duct (arrow). Used with permission. Lefkowitch JH, et al. *Gastroenterology* 1993; 104: 595–603.

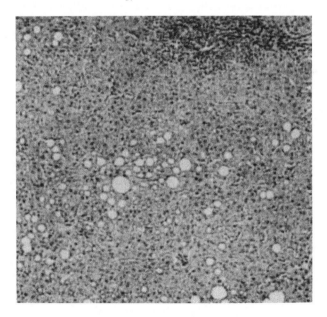

Figure 10.2 Mild large droplet fat in hepatocytes in chronic hepatitis C (H&E; original magnification × 100). Used with permission. Lefkowitch JH, et al. *Gastroenterology* 1993; 104: 595–603.

and/or lobular activity gives a very characteristic pathological appearance for HCV.[7]

It is important to be able to distinguish autoimmune hepatitis (AIH) from hepatitis due to HCV. Biopsies from AIH subjects tend to have more advanced findings such as bridging necrosis or cirrhosis. Plasma cells are abundant in the periportal inflammatory infiltrate and clusters of periportal liver cells organize into rosettes.[9]

The same staging system of liver biopsies is used in chronic hepatitis B and C (Chapter 5). In chronic hepatitis of any type, *chronic persistent hepatitis* is usually considered a non-progressive entity while *chronic active hepatitis* is thought a progressive entity. Whether this classification holds true is examined in the next section on natural history.

Natural History

Since hepatitis C appears largely to be an asymptomatic disease, the best understanding of the development of chronicity has come from prospectively followed transfusion associated cases. In such a setting, 40–60% of acute PT-NANB or hepatitis C cases develop chronic infection.[10-12]

Chronic infection is usually defined as a persistently elevated ALT value of greater than two and one half times normal for more than six months.[11] The time period of six months was borrowed from acute hepatitis B where it is well documented that spontaneous resolution seldom occurs after that interval. Six months may not be the optimal time division for hepatitis C chronicity.

In a U. S. Army study, 16 patients with PT-NANB had raised ALT values for six months but only ten were still elevated at one year.[13] A study of liver biopsies during acute NANB hepatitis showed resolution of ALT values in five patients within six months; however, two patients took ten and 16 months to normalize aminotransferase values.[14] Kiyosawa followed 70 patients with acute PT-NANB. 46 patients had an elevated ALT for six months but only 32 were still elevated after 12 months.[15] It is interesting to note all three of the foregoing studies have the same resolution rate of 30 to 38% in the period of six to twelve months after acute PT-NANB.

Spontaneous resolution beyond twelve months appears unusual. In the Sentinel county study of 85 anti-HCV positive patients (verified with HCV-RNA) followed for six years, two lost HCV antibody; one became negative at 45 months and the other at six years for an antibody loss of 0.6% per year.[11] A Japanese study followed 111 patients for an average of 8.8 years with four becoming EIA-1 negative (confirmed by

RIBA-II). The rate of natural loss of HCV was calculated to be 0.4% per year.[16] An early NIH study followed twelve patients with PT-NANB with elevated ALT values for more than 12 months. Four patients had sustained normalization of ALT results over a period of an additional one to three years. It is uncertain how many of these cases were due to hepatitis C since serology was not available.[17] Thus, it is likely that twelve months of elevated ALT values and the presence of hepatitis C antibody should be used for the definition of chronicity.[12]

Early studies of cirrhosis upon presentation indicated a rate of 10–20%.[12] Later studies, which may have less selection bias, report the prevalence of cirrhosis to be on the order of 0–3% (combined 3/220 or 1.4%).[1,11,14,20] To illustrate the bias involved in a referral population, a Stanford study of patients with chronic hepatitis C sent to their Liver Clinic showed a 46% rate of cirrhosis upon initial biopsy.[21]

>> *In the following sections on natural history, patients were either selected for their first liver biopsy or, as in most cases, only a portion of cases on follow-up were chosen for biopsy. In either case, a significant bias has been introduced in favor of progressive, or more severe disease, being reported. Thus, the natural history of hepatitis C will appear more ominous than it is in reality.*

Will a single liver biopsy accurately represent the stage of disease throughout the liver? That is, can disease activity vary among individual segments of the liver? No report has focused on chronic hepatitis C exclusively, but a routine second pass in 100 randomized patients with chronic hepatitis changed the histological stage only three times; three patients with chronic active hepatitis were reclassified as having cirrhosis on the second biopsy.[22] Another trial of percutaneous versus laparoscopic sampling of both liver lobes gave a 95% concordance rate.[23] Thus, sampling error does not appear to be a significant problem in patients with chronic hepatitis.

Chronic persistent hepatitis (newer term: "mild hepatitis")

Chronic persistent hepatitis (CPH) (Figure 5.1) is a histological stage of chronic HCV infection which lacks either piecemeal necrosis or fibrosis. In other diseases, such as autoimmune hepatitis or chronic hepatitis B, it is considered a non-progressive lesion; that is, it will not go on to cirrhosis.[24] Figure 10.3 reviews those reports which have performed

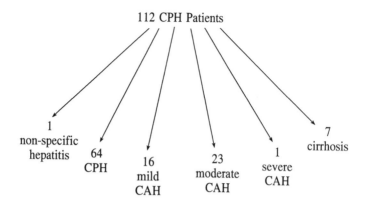

Figure 10.3 Follow-up of chronic persistent hepatitis. Compiled from references 16, 25–28.

follow-up liver biopsies on patients with CPH.[16,25–28] The time frames of follow-up are reported differently and do not allow an average time of observation to be calculated.

Most patients with CPH (65/112, 58%) do not progress to a worse histological picture. One patient improved to a non-specific reactive hepatitis picture. A smaller proportion (24/112, 21%) appear to progress to some degree of moderate or severe chronic active hepatitis. A small minority (7/112, 6%) result in cirrhosis after 5–32 years.

Chronic active hepatitis (newer term: "moderate hepatitis")

The presence of piecemeal necrosis defines the histological picture of chronic active hepatitis (CAH). If bridging necrosis spans from portal triad to portal triad, then a *severe* form of chronic active hepatitis is present. The following discussion does not include "mild" chronic active hepatitis; only two cases have been reported by the NIH and histology remained unchanged for these two on a later biopsy.

Figure 10.4 tabulates the reported cases of moderate CAH that have had follow-up liver biopsies.[16,26–30] Of 56 cases of "moderate" CAH, 6 improved to CPH, 22 stayed the same and 28 (50%) worsened to severe CAH or cirrhosis. Figure 10.4 tabulates the follow-up of severe CAH.[26] Of 25 cases, nine stayed the same and 16 progressed to cirrhosis.

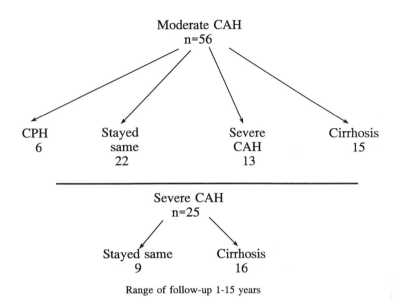

Range of follow-up 1-15 years

Figure 10.4 Follow-up pf chronic active hepatitis. Compiled from references 16, 26–30.

Progression

To summarize the prior sections on follow-up of histology, it appears that in the majority of cases CPH does not progress. Moderate CAH progresses 50% of the time to more severe forms and severe CAH usually progresses to cirrhosis. One case of CPH improved and 6 (11%) of moderate CAH actually improved their histology. The time span of the foregoing observations most often are on the order of two to ten years. CPH cases have been noted to stay unchanged for 14 to 18 years.[15] Follow-up for time periods less than ten years is probably too limited to appreciate the true incidence of cirrhosis or liver failure.[29] Commonly, the development of cirrhosis appears to take ten to twenty years or more. Cirrhosis due to chronic HCV is an indolent disease and largely asymptomatic until liver failure occurs. Cirrhosis caused by hepatitis C is surprisingly well tolerated compared to that from other causes. In a review by Harvey Alter, 20–25% of patients with PT-NANB related cirrhosis eventually sustain a liver-related fatality.[12]

On the other hand, occasional cases (n = 9) of rapidly developing cirrhosis in one to five years after a clearly defined risk factor for acquisition of HCV are reported.[27, 28, 30] Two conditions, hypogammaglobulinemia and HIV infection have been associated with rapid development of cirrhosis in chronic HCV infection[27,30] (Chapter 11).

An 18 year case-control study of 568 patients with PT-NANB hepatitis acquired in the 1970's has been reported.[10] The frequency of death from all causes among the hepatitis patients (resolved or chronic) was identical to that of a carefully matched group in whom hepatitis did not develop. The frequencies of cirrhosis (1.4% vs 1%) and hepatocellular carcinoma (0.2% vs 0.2%) were the same in the study and control group. However, the frequency of death (3.4%) from liver disease was higher in the hepatitis group than in the control group. In addition, deaths from liver disease increased at a slow but steady pace over time, suggesting that surviving patients with chronic infection may yet die of liver disease.[10, 29]

A caveat in interpreting the current data on the natural history of hepatitis C is that most of the literature reports cases acquired from transfusion associated sources; whether this mode of acquisition is truly representative of HCV acquired in other ways is unknown.

Summary of natural history

A majority of patients with chronic active hepatitis C tolerate their disease very well and do not appear to have progressive disease in time intervals of up to twenty years. A smaller subset of patients are identified with a histological picture of chronic active hepatitis that in more severe forms is predictably progressive. Progression of chronic active hepatitis is not inexorable since a few patients may improve their histological condition on follow-up. The exact proportions of the groups that will progress or remain stable have not been accurately determined. As pointed out previously, all series have a selection bias inherent in the design and likely describe chronic HCV as more aggressive than it probably is in reality.

The author believes that histology is a valuable predictor of progression. The classification of chronic persistent versus chronic active is used in the current text but these terms have recently been changed to "mild or severe hepatitis" (Chapter 5). It is true that outcomes may not be as predictable as in other types of chronic hepatitis; still, until better virological markers become available, the distinction should be retained.

The use of alcohol is poorly accounted for in all studies. The author notes that cirrhosis due to hepatitis C in young patients is invariably accompanied by regular, though not necessarily "excessive," use of alcohol. Alcohol use has been shown to accelerate progression of disease more often in both hepatitis B and C.[18,19] The HCV virus mutates more frequently with alcohol exposure and this could possibly lead to increased virulence or hepatocellular carcinoma.[31] Most of the deaths due to liver disease in the large NIH follow-up study seemed to be related to a history of alcoholism.[10] Future studies on natural history should categorize patients as to the amount of alcohol used before and during follow-up for HCV disease.

In conclusion, it seems that a majority of chronic hepatitis C patients have an indolent and benign course. A significant proportion, however, have progressive liver disease and it is this latter group that physicians need to identify and refer for liver biopsy and treatment with alfa-interferon as outlined in chapter nine.

Complications of Chronic HCV Infection

The reported association of a positive EIA-1 HCV test and hepatocellular carcinoma (HCC) ranges from 51% to 94%.[32, 33] HCC is proven to occur in hepatitis B (chapter five). The serological association of HCV with HCC persists in ranges above 50% even when patients who are positive for any marker of hepatitis B are removed. In contrast to hepatitis B where HCC may occur without cirrhosis being present, virtually all cases of HCC associated with HCV occur in the presence of cirrhosis.[32,34,35] As in hepatitis B, alcohol use has been associated with an accelerated appearance and increased incidence of HCC. Figure 10.5 compares the cumulative rate of HCC in cirrhosis due to alcohol or HCV and the combined risk factor group.[36] A Japanese study of 21 patients with NANB hepatitis (94% EIA-1 HCV positive), shows a time interval of 29 years (± 13.2) for the development of HCC after blood transfusion. Three cases took as long as 50 to 60 years to develop.[33]

Table 10.1   The development of hepatocellular carcinoma in Japanese patients with cirrhosis due to alcoholism, HCV or combined disease. Data derived from Yamauchi M, et al. Prevalence of hepatocellular carcinoma in patients with alcoholic cirrhosis and prior exposure to hepatitis C. *Am J Gastroenterology* 1993; 88:39–43.

	Alcoholic Cirrhosis Alone	HCV Cirrhosis Alone	HCV & Alcoholic Cirrhosis
3 Year	0	7.3%	13.3%
5 Year	8.3%	23.1%	41.3%
10 Year	18.5%	56.5%	80.7%

HCV-RNA has been demonstrated both in tumor and non-tumorous areas of livers afflicted with HCC and HCV.[34] If there is a direct causation of HCC by the hepatitis C virus, the mechanism of oncogenesis is not understood. HCV is an RNA virus that does not have reverse transcriptase activity; therefore, viral integration of HCV into host hepatocytic DNA cannot occur as it does in hepatitis B.[36] No DNA intermediates of HCV have been detected.[34] It is hypothesized that HCV, rather than directly transforming hepatocytes, may affect cell growth or differentiation indirectly by activating growth factors, oncogenes or DNA binding proteins.[34]

One study has shown a significant decrease in median survival of HCC when HCV is present (4 months vs 20 months).[35] If hepatectomy can be performed on the HCC, however, the five year survival for HCC is independent of HCV status.[32]

It is not clear if patients who are coinfected with both HBV and HCV experience synergism in the risk for HCC. One study did not show any clinical differences in HCC between coinfected and single infection with either HBV or HCV.[37]

Further work needs to be done to elucidate the mechanism of HCC development in HCV disease and associated factors beyond alcohol use.

Essential mixed cryoglobulinemia

Essential mixed cryoglobulinemia (EMC) is a disorder characterized by the clinical triad of purpura, arthralgia and weakness. Vasculitis can occur with involvement of kidneys, nerves or brain. The diagnosis is based on finding serum cryoglobulins consisting of polyclonal IgG and monoclonal IgM proteins.[38]

A high frequency of hepatitis B surface antigen and antibody in serum and cryoprecipitates from patients with EMC has been reported; however, others have failed to find any marker of hepatitis B in most patients.[39] The association between hepatitis B and EMC remains controversial. When EMC patients are tested for HCV in the serum with EIA-2, studies have reported a 42 to 96% prevalence. Further, the prevalence of EIA-2 in cryoprecipitates may be as high as 96%.[40, 41]

EIA-2 may underestimate the prevalence of HCV in EMC. Agrello, et al, report a 42% occurrence of EIA-2 but an 84% prevalence of HCV-RNA in serum.[40] Reversing the question, only one report has looked at the prevalence of elevated cryoglobulins in chronic HCV patients. Cacoub et al. found 17% (22/127) to have elevated cryoglobulins of the EMC type but only 6% (7/107) to have clinical symptoms related to EMC.[42]

A high correlation of HCV in patients with EMC does not prove a causal relationship. Treatment of patients with EMC and HCV with alfa-interferon has yielded additional information. Casaril, et al, report negativization of the cryocrit in seven patients who responded to alfa-interferon. In non-responders, no change occurred in the cryoglobulin level.[43] In a second study, the manifestations of cryoglobulinemia disappeared in two patients who had a sustained normalization of aminotransferases 15 months after cessation of α-interferon.[44] Response to alfa-interferon would seem to provide proof that HCV causes EMC; however, reduction in cryoglobulinemia occurs in a variety of diseases (e.g., cancer, multiple myeloma) when alfa-interferon is given.[45]

Thus, it is likely that HCV is involved in some manner as a cause or promoter of EMC. Final proof awaits better understanding of the pathogenesis of EMC or the isolation of the hepatitis C virus.

Porphyria cutanea tarda

Porphyria cutanea tarda (PCT), the most common form of porphyria worldwide, is caused by the reduced activity of the hepatic enzyme uroporphyrinogen decarboxyloase (URO-D). PCT is manifested by the development of cutaneous vesicles in sun-exposed areas. Increased skin fragility, bruising, hypertrichosis and hyperpigmentation can occur.[46]

PCT is thought to be an acquired defect in most cases but is rarely inherited as an autosomal trait. Alcohol abuse, estrogen use and iron overload may be causative factors since withdrawal of the agent or phlebotomy causes clinical improvement.[47] Liver disease is very common in patients with PCT.[48]

Three reports of large groups of PCT patients in southern Europe have reported a prevalence of RIBA-II HCV positivity ranging from 62 to 82%.[46, 48, 49] There are no reports of the effects of alfa-interferon on the course of the HCV virus in PCT patients or its effect on the activity of the URO-D enzyme.

The group with the first report on the association of PCT and HCV, Fargion, et al., have a follow-up study showing an HCV prevalence of 82% (RIBA-II), alcohol abuse in 40% and iron overload in 45%. These investigators emphasize the multifactorial nature of PCT.[49]

Miscellaneous conditions

Lichen planus (LP) is a skin disorder manifested by an eruption of papules (lichen) which are flat (planus). The violaceous, scaling, pruritic papules are characteristically found on flexor surfaces, mucous membranes or genitalia. It is hypothesized to have a cell-mediated autoimmune basis.[51] LP and HCV occurring together in the same patients are reported.[52,53] Liver biopsies performed in five patients with LP showed chronic active hepatitis in all five.[54] A survey in France of 61 consecutive patients with chronic active hepatitis due to HCV showed a five percent prevalence of LP.[54] Exacerbation of LP during alfa-interferon treatment for HCV and amelioration after cessation of treatment has been noted.[55]

Autoimmune diseases such as systemic lupus erythematosus, Wegener's granulomatosis and the lymphocytic sialoadenitis of Sjögrens syndrome do *not* appear related to HCV.[56,57] An association between periarteritis nodosa and hepatitis C appears doubtful.[58]

Aplastic anemia is associated with the presence of non-A, non-B hepatitis.[59] However, extensive investigation with hepatitis C markers seems to rule out HCV as a significant cause.[60,61] It is likely that other unidentified viruses may be responsible.

The occurrence of Mooren's corneal ulcers (peripheral corneal eye ulcers) in two patients with positive HCV-RNA has been reported. Alfa-interferon therapy caused marked improvement in these two patients who were refractory to customary treatment.[62]

Clinical Evaluation

Due to the large number of patients who test positive for hepatitis C, primary care physicians need a protocol for determining which patients should be referred to a liver specialist. Obviously, patients need a history, physical examination and serological liver tests. The object of the clinical evaluation is to determine if the patient has significant liver damage or a progressive condition that will result in significant liver damage. The presence or absence of these conditions, along with other factors, help to determine eligibility for alfa-interferon treatment (Chapter 12).

Physical findings indicative of progressive liver disease include spider nevi, palmar erythema and a palpable liver which is firm on examination.[64]

Three laboratory features, serum albumin, alanine aminotransferase (ALT), and platelet count, may indicate those patients with progressive disease. All laboratory values need to be evaluated in context of the entire picture; that is, reliance upon a single parameter can be misleading. In an otherwise healthy patient, hypoalbuminemia is a sign of significant liver disease, however, patients with early cirrhosis may have normal albumin values.

A low platelet count, defined as less than 140,000 cells cc^3, reflects hypersplenism secondary to portal hypertension and is fairly specific (52%) and sensitive (96%) for significant liver disease in the absence of other obvious causes of thrombocytopenia.[64]

An elevated ALT value, particularly above 200 IU/L (5 × normal), is predictive of piecemeal necrosis and chronic active hepatitis (CAH).[65] However, reliance on a single ALT value less than 200 IU/L does not exclude significant liver disease. ALT values in hepatitis C are known to fluctuate dramatically. In one study of three consecutive ALT results in the same patient, 21% of patients with ALT ≤ 2x normal had CAH and 20% of patients with ALT ≥ 5 × normal had chronic persistent hepatitis.[65]

It is known that as cirrhosis approaches, ALT values tend to regress back towards the normal range and AST values stay the same or increase slightly. Thus, the AST/ALT ratio is less than one for non-cirrhotic disease and greater than one in cirrhosis.[66]

In those patients who present without signs of advanced liver disease, two options exist for defining whether or not progressive liver disease is present. A liver biopsy may be done or the patient may be followed prospectively over time and examined periodically. Some in the field of hepatitis C advocate that all patients with a true positive HCV test undergo a liver biopsy.[63] The arguments against biopsing everyone with asymptomatic disease are: one, only a minority of patients with chronic HCV appear to have progressive disease; two, if 1.8% of the population is infected with HCV (CDC, unpublished), the economic costs of such a recommendation are staggering; and three, liver biopsy has a low but definite risk of morbidity or mortality.

The argument in favor of biopsing every hepatitis C patient is that a few cases of advanced histological lesions have been reported with normal or near normal ALT values.[63,65] Turning the question around, Esteban, et al., report that all HCV patients with a normal liver biopsy have a normal ALT value.[67] Brillant, et al.[68] have followed four symptom-free individuals with positive HCV-RNA tests but normal ALT values for three years. Liver biopsies remained normal.

However, when hepatitis C does progress, it usually does so slowly and an instantaneous decision (i.e., an immediate liver biopsy) is not mandatory. Those patients who are not biopsied should be seen at least yearly with a review of their physical exam and liver tests. Deterioration of test results or the onset of symptoms can then lead to a liver biopsy on follow-up.

Treatment Summary of Hepatitis C

1. Hepatitis C is defined as a chronic infection after being present for six to twelve months.
2. Referral for possible liver biopsy and alfa-interferon treatment (Chapter 12) depends on the degree of liver damage and the clinical situation. Parameters of progressive liver disease include:
   - physical examination (spider nevi, palmar erythema, etc.)
   - the degree of ALT abnormality (Undue reliance on a mildly elevated ALT to exclude significant liver disease can be misleading. The AST/ALT ratio should also be examined [see text]).
   - serum albumin
   - platelet count
3. Patients with mild liver disease (i.e., absence of findings suggestive of progressive liver disease) may also be candidates for referral. Patients in the following categories should particularly be encouraged to seek further evaluation:
   - those with symptoms of fatigue
   - those with anxiety over the variable prognosis of chronic hepatitis C
   - health care workers
   - women who may become pregnant
4. Complications of HCV infection include:
   - hepatocellular carcinoma (after cirrhosis occurs)
   - essential mixed cryoglobulinemia
   - porphyria cutanea tarda
   - lichen planus
   - Mooren's corneal ulcer (tentative)
   - some types of glomerulonephritis (tentative—see Chapter 12)

References

1. McCaughan GW, McGuiness PH, Bishop GA, et al. Clinical assessment and incidence of hepatitis C RNA in 50 consecutive RIBA-positive volunteer blood donors. *Med J Aust* 1992; 157:231–233.

2. Dienstag JL. Non-A, non-B hepatitis. I. Recognition, epidemiology, and clinical features. *Gastroenterology* 1983; 85:439–462.
3. Alter HJ, Purcell RH, Feinstone SM, et al. Non-A, non-B hepatitis: a review and interim report of an ongoing prospective study. In: Szmuners W, Alter HJ, Maynard JE, eds. *Viral hepatitis: 1981 international symposium.* Philadelphia: Franklin Institute Press, 1982: 359–369.
4. Sampliner RE, Woronow DI, Alter MJ, et al. Community-acquired non-A, non-B hepatitis: clinical characteristics and chronicity. *J Med Vir* 1984; 13:125–130.
5. Merican I, Sherlock S, McIntyre N, et al. Clinical, biochemical and histological features in 102 patients with chronic hepatitis C virus infection. *Quart J Med* 1993; 86:119–125.
6. Lefkowitch JH, Schiff ER, Davis GL, et al. Pathological diagnosis of chronic hepatitis C: a multicenter comparative study with chronic hepatitis B. *Gastroenterology* 1993; 104:595–603.
7. Scheuer PJ, Ashrafzadeh P, Sherlock S, et al. The pathology of hepatitis C. *Hepatology* 1992; 15:567–571.
8. Areias J, Pedroto I, Motos P, et al. Bile duct changes of chronic hepatitis C are not associated with abnormalities of serum alkaline phosphatase. *Hepatology* 1993; 18:222 (abstract).
9. Bach N, Thung SN, Schaffner F. The histological features of chronic hepatitis C and autoimmune chronic hepatitis: a comparative analysis. *Hepatology* 1992; 15:572–577.
10. Seeff LB, Buskell-Bales Z, Wright EC, et al. Long-term mortality after transfusion-associated non-A, non-B hepatitis. *N Engl J Med* 1992; 327:1906–1911.
11. Alter MJ, Margolis HS, Krawczynski K, et al. The natural history of community-acquired hepatitis C in the United States. *N Engl J Med* 1992; 327:1899–1905.
12. Alter HJ. Chronic consequences of non-A, non-B hepatitis. In: Seeff LB, Lewis JH, eds. *Current Perspectives in Hepatology.* New York. Plenum, 1989.
13. Knodell RG, Conrad NE, Ishak KG. Development of chronic liver disease after acute non-A, non-B post-transfusion hepatitis: role of gamma globulin prophylaxis in its prevention. *Gastroenterology* 1977; 72:902–909.
14. Realdi G, Alberti A, Rugge M, et al. Long-term follow-up of acute and chronic non-A, non-B post-transfusion hepatitis: evidence of progression to liver cirrhosis. *Gut* 1982: 23:270–575.

15. Kiyosawa K, Akahane Y, Nagata A, et al. The significance of blood transfusion in non-A, non-B chronic liver disease in Japan. *Vox Sang* 1982; 43:45–52.

16. Yousuf M, Nakano E, Tanaka T, et al. Persistence of viremia in patients with type-C chronic hepatitis during long-term follow-up. *Scand J Gastroenterology* 1992; 27:812–816.

17. Berman M, Alter HJ, Ishak KG, et al. The chronic sequelae of non-A, non-B hepatitis. *Ann Intern Med* 1979; 91:1–6.

18. Shiomi S, Kuroki T, Minamitani S, et al. Effect of drinking on the outcome of cirrhosis with hepatitis B or C. *J Gast Hepat* 1992; 7:274–276.

19. Caldwell SH, Li X, Rourk RM, et al. Hepatitis C infection by polymerase chain reaction in alcoholics: false positive ELISA results and the influence of infection on a clinical prognostic score. *Am J Gastroenterology* 1992; 88:1016–1021.

20. Donato MF, Ronchi G, Callea F, et al. Long-term follow-up of anti-HCV positive chronic persistent hepatitis. *Hepatology* 1992; 16:201 (abstract).

21. Ladenheim J, Martin MC, Gregory PB, et al. Natural history of chronic hepatitis C: baseline characteristics and correlation between laboratory tests and liver biopsy findings. *Gastroenterology* 1993; 104:1021 (abstract).

22. Papini E, Pacella CM, Rossi Z, et al. A randomized trial of ultrasound guided anterior subcostal liver biopsy versus the conventional Menghini technique. *J Hepatology* 1992; 13:291–297.

23. Picciotto A, Ciravegna G, Lapertosa G, et al. Percutaneous or laparoscopic needle biopsy in the evaluation of chronic liver disease? *Am J Gastroenterology* 1984; 79:567–568.

24. Chronic hepatitis. In: Sherlock S, Dooley J. *Disease of the Liver and Biliary System*, London: Blackwell Scientific Publishers, 1993: 293–321.

25. Donato MF, Ronchi G, Callea F, et al. Long-term follow-up study of anti-HCV positive chronic persistent hepatitis. *Hepatology* 1992; 16:201 (astract).

26. Takahashi M, Yamada G, Miyamoto R, et al. Natural course of chronic hepatitis C. *Am J Gastroenterology* 1993; 88:240–243.

27. Mattsson L, Weiland O, Glaumann H. Long-term follow-up of chronic post-transfusion non-A, non-B hepatitis: clinical and histological outcome. *Liver* 1988; 8:184–188.

28. Di Bisceglie AM, Goodman ZD, Ishak KG, et al. Long-term clinical and histopathological follow-up of chronic post-transfusion hepatitis. *Hepatology* 1991; 14:969–974.

29. Czaja AJ. Chronic hepatitis C virus infection—a disease in waiting? *N Engl J Med* 1992; 327:1949–1950.

30. Martin P, Di Bisceglie AM, Kassianides C, et al. Rapidly progressive non-A, non-B hepatitis in patients with human immunodeficiency virus infection. *Gastroenterology* 1989; 97:1559–1561.

31. Coelho-little E, Jeffers LJ, Uchman S, et al. HCV exhibits a higher degree of mutability in patients with a background of alcohol abuse. *Gastroenterology* 1993; 104:901 (abstract).

32. Takeda S, Nagafuchi Y, Tashiro H, et al. Anti-hepatitis C virus status in hepatocellular carcinoma and the influence on clinicopathological findings and operative results. *Br J Surg* 1992; 79:1195–1198.

33. Kiyosawa K, Sodeyama T, Tanaka E, et al. Interrelationship of blood transfusions, non-A, non-B hepatitis and hepatocellular carcinoma: analysis by detection of antibody to hepatitis C virus. *Hepatology* 1990; 12:671–675.

34. Gerber MA, Shieh YS, Shim KS, et al. Detection of replicative hepatitis C virus sequences in hepatocellular carcinoma. *Am J Path* 1992; 141:1271–1277.

35. Farinati F, Fagiuoli S, DeMaria N, et al. Anti-HCV positive hepatocellular carcinoma in cirrhosis. *J Hepatology* 1992; 14:183–187.

36. Yamauchi M, Nakahara M, Maezawa Y, et al. Prevalence of hepatocellular carcinoma in patients with alcoholic cirrhosis and prior exposure to hepatitis C. *Am J Gastroenterology* 1993; 88:39–43.

37. Ruiz J, Sangro B, Cuende JI, et al. Hepatitis B and C viral infections in patients with hepatocellular carcinoma. *Hepatology* 1992; 16:637–641.

38. Misiani R, Bellavita P, Fenili D, et al. Hepatitis C virus infection in patients with essential mixed cryoglobulinemia. *Ann Intern Med* 1992; 117:573–577.

39. Popp JW Jr, Dienstag JL, Wands JR, et al. Essential mixed cryoglobulinemia without evidence for hepatitis B virus infection. *Ann Intern Med* 1980; 92:379–383.

40. Agnello V, Chung RT, Kaplan LM. A role for hepatitis C infection in type II cryoglobulinemia. *N Engl J Med* 1992; 327:1490–1495.

41. Misiani R, Bellavita P, Riuniti O, et al. Hepatitis C virus and cryoglobulinemia. *N Engl J Med* 1992; 328:1121.

42. Cacoub P, Lunel F, Musset L, et al. Hepatitis C virus and cryoglobulinemia. *N Engl J Med* 1993; 328:1121–1122.

43. Casaril M, Capra F, Tognella P, et al. Cryoglobulinemia and HCV chronic hepatitis: effects of alpha IFN therapy. *J Hepatology* 1992; 16 (Suppl 1):S-84.

44. Castilla A, Castilla I, Prieto J. α-Interferon therapy for hepatitis C virus chronic infection with mixed cryoglobulinemia. *Am J Gastroenterology* 1993; 88:466–467.

45. Bibas M, Andriani A. Hepatitis C virus and cryoglobulinemia. *N Engl J Med* 1993; 328:1123.

46. Fargion S, Piperno A, Cappellini MD, et al. Hepatitis C virus and porphyria cutanea tarda: evidence of a strong association. *Hepatology* 1992; 16:1322–1326.

47. Cutaneous hepatitis porphyria: porphyria cutanea tarda and symptomatic porphyria. In: Moore MR, McColl KE, Rimington C, et al, eds. *Disorders of porphyria metabolism.* New York: Plenum, 1987: 179–200.

48. Herrero C, Vicenta A, Bruguera M, et al. Is hepatitis C virus infection a trigger of porphyria cutanea tarda? *Lancet* 1993; 341:788–789.

49. De Castro M, Sanchez J, Herrera JF, et al. Hepatitis C virus antibodies and liver disease in patients with porphyria cutanea tarda. *Hepatology* 1993; 17:551–557.

50. Fargion S, Piperno A, Fracanzani AL, et al. Multifactorial pathogenesis of liver disease in patients with porphyria cutanea tarda. *Hepatology* 1992; 16:231 (abstract).

51. Arndt KA. Lichen planus. In: Fitzpatrick TB, Eisen AZ, Wolff K, et al. *Dermatology in general medicine.* 3rd edition. New York: McGraw-Hill, 1987: 967–968.

52. Agner T, Fogh H, Weismann K. The relation between lichen planus and hepatitis C: a case report. *Acta Derm Venereaol* (Stockh) 1992; 72:380.

53. Rebora A, Robert E, Rongioletti F. Clinical and laboratory presentation of lichen planus patients with chronic liver disease. *J Derm Sci* 1992; 4:38–41.

54. Jubert C, Pawlotsky JM, Pouget F, et al. Lichen planus and hepatitis C virus-related chronic active hepatitis. *Arch Dermatol* 1994; 130:73–76.

55. Protzer U, Ochsendorf FR, Leopolder-Ochsendorf A, et al. Exacerbation of lichen planus during interferon alfa-2a therapy for chronic active hepatitis C. *Gastroenterology* 1993; 104:903–905.

56. Pawlotsky JM, BenYahia M, Andre C, et al. Immunological disorders associated with C viral chronic hepatitis: a prospective evaluation. *Hepatology* 1992; 16:217 (abstract).

57. Cacoub P, Lunel-Fabiani F, Du LT. Polyarteritis nodosa and hepatitis C infection. *Ann Intern Med* 1992; 116:605.

58. Deny P, Guillevin L, Bonacorsi S, et al. Association between hepatitis C virus and polyarteritis nodosa. *Clin Exp Rheu* 1992; 10:319.

59. Zeldis JB, Dienstag JL, Gale RP. Aplastic anemia and non-A, non-B hepatitis. *Am J Med* 1983; 74:64–68.

60. Pol S, Thiers V, Driss F, et al. HCV plays no role in hepatitis-associated aplastic anemia. *Hepatology* 1992; 16:71 (abstract).

61. Hibbs JR, Frickhofen N, Rosenfeld SJ, et al. Aplastic anemia and viral hepatitis: Non-A, non-B, non-C? *JAMA* 1992; 267:2051–2054.

62. Wilson SE, Lee WM, Murakami C, et al. Mooren's corneal ulcers and hepatitis C virus infection. *N Engl J Med* 1993; 329:62.

63. Alberti A, Morsica G, Chemello L, et al. Hepatitis C viraemia and liver disease in symptom-free individuals with anti-HCV. *Lancet* 1992; 340:697–698.

64. Tine F, Caltagirone M, Camma C, et al. Clinical indicants of compensated cirrhosis: a prospective study. In: Dianzani MU, Gentilini P. *Chronic Liver Damage.* New York: Elsevier-Science, 1990:187–198.

65. Haber MM, West AB, Reuben A. Relationship of alanine aminotransferase to histologic findings in chronic hepatitis C. *Gastroenterology* 1993; 104:A912 (abstract).

66. Williams AL, Hoofnagle JH. Ratio of serum aspartate to alanine aminotransferase in chronic hepatitis. *Gastroenterology* 1988; 95:734–739.

67. Esteban JI, Lopez-Talavera JC, Genesca J, et al. Evaluation of anti-HCV positive blood donors identified during routine screening. *Arch Virol (Suppl)* 1992; 4:244–246.

68. Brillanti S, Foli M, Gaiani S, et al. Persistent hepatitis C viraemia without liver disease. *Lancet* 1993; 341:464–465.

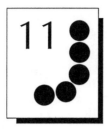

Special Topics in Hepatitis C

Prevention
Pediatrics
Pregnancy
Renal Disease
Coinfection with HCV and HIV

Prevention of Non-A, Non-B Hepatitis (Hepatitis C) by Gamma Globulin

Since gamma globulin (ISG) has been shown to be helpful in prevention of secondary cases due to hepatitis A or B, the use of ISG for prevention of non-A, non-B (type C) hepatitis has also undergone intense scrutiny.

Seventeen trials of gamma globulin to prevent post-transfusion hepatitis of any type have been reported.[1, 2] Most were done in the era before hepatitis A and B testing and thus have uncertain applicability now. In addition, the way in which ISG is prepared has been modified since 1972.[3] Six trials have been published since 1976 and these will be reviewed. Five controlled studies have looked at the prevention of NANB hepatitis from transfusion; two trials do not show any reduction in incidence of NANB hepatitis;[1, 4] however, three trials show a significant reduction in the incidence of transfusion associated NANB hepatitis.[3, 5, 6] The principle difference in outcome of these trials is

179

ably related to the timing of gamma globulin injection. In the three trials in which ISG proved efficacious, ISG was given prior to the blood products, and in the two trials where ISG proved ineffective, the ISG was started after transfusions were received.

A sixth trial reviewed the incidence of all types of viral hepatitis in U.S. soldiers serving in Korea from 1967 to 1970. 107,803 soldiers received either ISG or placebo upon arrival and before exposure. Only 28 patients developed NANB hepatitis. A significant reduction of NANB hepatitis occurred in those soldiers developing hepatitis in the first six months of ISG injection (ISG 2, placebo 14); but in those failing to receive a follow-up shot at six months, no difference was seen in the incidence of NANB hepatitis beyond six months of the first shot (ISG 5, placebo7).[7]

Pre-exposure prophylaxis, then, may offer a degree of protection against the development of NANB hepatitis. In regards to transfusion related NANB hepatitis, the issue is moot since donor blood screening has reduced the occurrence of hepatitis C to extremely low levels compared to the 8–25% incidence cited in prior studies on transfusion associated hepatitis.

The U.S. Army study in Korea injected 107,000 soldiers and reduced the occurrence of NANB by 14 cases. ISG is now made differently and whether this trial supports the use of pre-exposure prophylaxis for non-transfusion associated prevention remains speculative.

The foregoing data on pre-exposure prophylaxis offers no support for post-exposure prophylaxis of hepatitis C. This is the more common question concerning hepatitis C where the role of ISG for prevention is often considered in needlestick incidents or obstetrical situations. Post-exposure use of ISG to prevent hepatitis C transmission may not work for three additional reasons. First, a neutralizing antibody for hepatitis C has not yet been discovered.[8] Secondly, the NIH studies of rechallenging chimpanzees who appear to resolve a prior hepatitis C episode show that protective immunity apparently does not develop. Ten challenges with the same or different strain of hepatitis C in five different chimpanzees resulted in the reappearance of HCV viremia every time.[9] The same phenomenon of recurrence of HCV infection in mulitply transfused thalassemic children has also been noted.[10] Third, a study which attempted to neutralize HCV by incubating the virus with plasma containing anti-HCV failed to prevent infection when this mixture was injected into chimpanzees.[8]

Furthermore, in many areas outside the United States (e. g., Canada), plasma collected for ISG use is screened for HCV antibody. Units which are HCV positive are not used for ISG preparation. Thus, ISG which is prepared from screened blood would be expected to contain little activity against hepatitis C.[11]

In summary, post-exposure prophylaxis has not been shown to be effective in preventing transfusion associated NANB hepatitis. Significant theoretical reasons and experimental data exists to suggest that neutralizing antibodies against hepatitis C may not exist. No agreement has been reached concerning post-exposure prophylaxis with ISG for needlesticks or perinatal exposure of hepatitis C.[2,12] At the current time, the author does not recommend ISG use for prevention of hepatitis C.

Pediatrics

Little is written about hepatitis C in children. Most reports have been from young patients who also have hemophilia, malignancy or end stage renal failure.[13-15] As in adults, hepatitis C appears to be an asymptomatic disease.[16] The pathology in a referral population of 16 children appears very similar to the types and proportions in the adult population.[17] Two cases of giant cell hepatitis in neonates have been reported where the children and their mothers were all RIBA-II positive.[18]

Limited information on the natural history of HCV infection in pediatrics suggests that the chronicity and long-term outcomes are similar to that seen in adults. 57% of multiply transfused beta-thalassemic children who experienced acute hepatitis C went on to chronicity.[19] In a twelve year follow-up, one of twelve children chronically infected cleared RIBA-II.[2] In a similar study with a mean follow-up of five years, one out of eleven developed persistently normal ALT values.[17]

Five patients with persistently elevated ALT have had a repeat biopsy two to eight years later. Histology was unchanged in all five cases: two maintained a mild CAH, two of CPH and one of minimal changes.[17]

No growth retardation occurs in chronic hepatitis C. Encephalopathy, ascites or bleeding did not develop in 16 HCV positive children followed for up to14 years.[17] As of this writing, the author is unaware of any child who has died due to liver disease caused solely by hepatitis C. The lack of cases is consistent with the observation in adults that when cirrhosis does occur, a time period of ten to twenty years or more is required (Chapter 10).

Only a few children have been treated with alfa-interferon. Twelve young patients with beta-thalassemia were treated for eight months with 5/12 (42%) gaining a sustained normalization of ALT values. Hemolytic anemia, a side effect of alfa-interferon not seen in adults, caused two patients to discontinue therapy at 7 and 8 weeks.[20] A second study of eleven children showed 36% to have normal ALT values at the end of six months of treatment but this percentage increased to 90% at fifteen months of follow-up. Thereafter, relapse occurred in five children for a sustained ALT normalization rate of 45% (5/11). Side effects were similar to those seen in the adult population. One patient was worsened by alfa-interferon and responded to immunosuppression suggesting auto-immune hepatitis mimicked hepatitis C infection.[21] This problem of mimicry is well known in adults (Chapter 9). Treatment of patients less than 18 years of age is currently not approved by the Food and Drug Administration in the United States.

In contrast to hepatitis B, the limited information available for the pediatric population does not suggest any major age-related difference in the course or outcome of HCV disease. Further information in this area is greatly needed.

Pregnancy

As in hepatitis A and B, the mother who has acute or chronic hepatitis C without cirrhosis does not experience an increased risk of congenital malformations, stillbirths, abortions, or intrauterine malnutrition.[22–24] One study shows an increase in prematurity from mothers with non-B hepatitis.[22] This may be due to the fact that mothers who are hepatitis C positive (RIBA-II) were seven times less likely to obtain pre-natal care than their non-HCV counterparts.[23]

Perinatal transmission appears to be less than 5% and is reviewed in Chapter 9. Gamma globulin for the prevention of perinatally acquired hepatitis C has not been studied and has no proven benefit (see prevention section earlier in chapter).

Since hepatitis C is *not* a cause of poor outcome in pregnant women, nor often transmitted perinatally, nor prevented by gamma globulin, prenatal screening of pregnant women for hepatitis C is not recommended.[23]

Breast milk appears not to be infected with hepatitis C. A Japanese study of ten mothers who were persistently HCV-RNA positive in serum showed no evidence of HCV-RNA in breast milk collected within five days of delivery and upon monthly followup. None of the ten infants showed HCV-RNA in the serum for up to ten months of followup.[25] This study confirms the lack of detection of HCV in breast milk performed by a Stanford group.[26]

Renal Disease

Does HCV cause kidney disease?

Hepatitis B has traditionally been the only hepatotrophic virus thought to cause intrinsic renal disease. Recently, RJ Johnson et al.[27] reported eight cases of membranoproliferative glomerulonephritis which were positive for EIA-2 and HCV-RNA. Five cases were also positive for cryoglobulins so whether this group is an independent group or a subset of essential mixed cryoglobulinemia with renal involvement is not clear. The authors were unable to identify HCV antigen or RNA in the glomerular lesions.

Two cases of membranous glomerulonephritis occurring with the onset of HCV infection in bone marrow transplants have been reported.[28] In these cases, PCR probes of kidney biopsy specimens showed the presence of HCV.

Reversing the question, 110 adult patients with primary glomerulonephritis in France were tested for HCV by RIBA-II and all were negative.[29] However, no cases of membranoproliferative glomerulonephritis were included in the French study. Renal disease, if it occurs at all, is seldom due to HCV infection. Further work needs to be done in this area.

HCV prevalence in dialysis units

The prevalence of second generation EIA or RIBA positive results in patients with end stage renal disease (ESRD) or undergoing transplantation ranges from 4.2% to 27%.[30,31]

Positivity for HCV has correlated with the number of blood transfusions received and the length of time on hemodialysis.[32,33] This has led to speculation as to whether HCV patients with ESRD on hemodialysis should be isolated in the same manner as patients with HBV and ESRD undergoing hemodialysis.[33] It is difficult to separate out the effect of blood transfusions from the length of time on dialysis since these risk factors are correlated. Two trends should help clarify the risk relationship between dialysis and HCV. Acquisition of hepatitis C through blood transfusions is now uncommon. Blood units screened by EIA 2 HCV and other surrogate markers have an infectivity rate of 0.03% per unit; that is, one in 3,000 units will transmit post-transfusion hepatitis. Secondly, the need for transfusion is being reduced by the use of erythopoietin.[34]

It is not clear whether hemodialysis by itself is a risk for acquiring HCV infection. In one study, sharing machines between HCV positive and negative patients was not a risk factor for becoming HCV positive. However, having an HCV positive neighbor during dialysis appeared to be a possible risk factor.[33]

A study in Naples, Italy isolated 22 HCV positive patients both by machine and area. The 57 patients who were HCV negative and dialyzed separately remained RIBA-II negative for the entire year of the study.[35]

A uniform policy regarding isolation of HCV positive patients has not been made in the United States. More data is needed. Studies should follow prospectively HCV negative ESRD patients starting on hemodialysis in those units who isolate patients compared to those who do not.

Impact of HCV infection upon renal transplantation

Pol et al., in the first large report of HCV upon the impact of renal transplantation, showed that HCV infection does not influence the survival of either patients or the renal allograft over one to twenty years (mean 4.3 years) (Figure 11.1).[36]

A Vanderbilt study by Ynares et al.[37] also demonstrates no difference in graft or patient survival with HCV status at both five and ten year follow-up. One patient required a simultaneous liver and kidney transplant ten years after the onset of liver disease due to HCV. Two patients with HCV died of liver failure but three patients in the HCV-negative group also died of liver failure.

Three HCV positive patients who had a renal transplant in a study from Madrid, Spain developed liver failure and required liver transplantation at 24, 48 and 120 months after renal transplantation. It is emphasized in the Spanish study that the three cases which developed liver failure occurred only in the renal allograft group which received azothioprine (3/23).[38] None of their 60 HCV positive patients receiving cyclosporine A developed liver failure.

Whether alfa-interferon can be used to treat renal transplant patients with HCV infection is unknown. The principle fear of using alfa-interferon in this setting is the possibility of causing organ rejection. The author is aware of a handful of unreported anecdotal cases where alfa-interferon was used in this situation. No organ rejection occurred but there was also no significant amelioration of the HCV disease.

Based upon the two large studies indicating that HCV does not affect the survival of the patient or the allograft for ten years, and in a

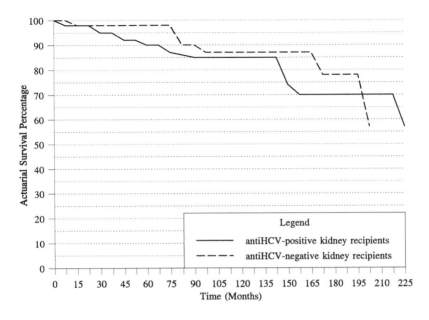

Figure 11.1 Actuarial survival curve of antiHCV-positive and antiHCV-negative kidney recipients. Number indicates the number of patients according to HCV status. Used by permission. Pol S, et al. Hepatitis C virus in kidney recipients. *J Hepatol* 1992; 15:202–6.

few cases to twenty years, it has been the author's practice not to screen HCV positive ESRD candidates for kidney transplantation with a liver biopsy unless they have overt manifestations of liver disease. In other words, the presence of HCV infection alone should not make a patient ineligible for renal transplantation.

In summary, HCV infection is prevalent in ESRD or renal transplant patients because of multiple blood transfusions, possible risk of hemodialysis and receipt of infected donor organs. No systematic data exists for the efficacy and side-effects of alfa-interferon in HCV patients with ESRD or renal allografts. The same statement also applies to other allografts such as heart, lung or bone marrow patients.

Coinfection with HCV and HIV

Eyster et al.[39] have followed 97 male hemophiliacs infected with HCV and HIV but not hepatitis B for up to 27 years after first receiving clotting concentrates. The majority of these patients were infected with HIV between 1978 and 1986, more than ten years after they were infected with HCV. Nine patients have developed decompensated liver disease as defined by the development of ascites, bleeding varices, hepatic encephalopathy or persistent hyperbilirubinemia. Six of the nine patients had received AZT, DDI or trimethoprim/sulfamethoxazole. In two patients, alcohol may have been a contributing factor. The outcome of dually infected patients compares unfavorably with their similar group of hemophiliacs who are HCV positive but HIV negative, where none of 59 patients developed decompensated liver disease over the same observation period.

Others have noted the rapid development of cirrhosis in a three to five year period after the onset of combined HCV/HIV infection.[40,41] At least two factors are likely to be responsible for more severe disease occurring in co-infected patients. First, HCV, in contrast to hepatitis B, is cytopathic rather than immunopathic and thus more cell damage occurs in HCV when immune suppression takes place.[42] Secondly, in a related way, HCV replication is noted to be increased in patients with HIV infection compared to those without.[41, 43]

The poorer outcome of coinfected patients is not a uniform experience. Areias, et al.,[44] in a Portugese study of combined infection in drug addicts did not find any significant difference between twelve co-infected patients versus thirty with HCV infection alone. The prevalence of cirrhosis in the two groups was about ten per cent.

Turning the question around, it is not clear if hepatitis C has a deleterious effect on the course of HIV disease. HIV viremia does not appear to be increased in HCV coinfections.[45]

The prevalence of human immunodeficiency virus seems to facilitate sexual transmission of the hepatitis C virus. A marked increase in the positivity of HCV was seen in sexual partners of dually infected patients versus partners of those patients who were only infected with HCV.[46] Dually infected pregnant women also seem to transmit HCV virus more frequently at the time of birth (Chapter 9).

Little data exist on the treatment of HCV with alfa-interferon in HIV positive patients. Boyer, et al.,[47] in a French study report treating twelve co-infected patients (two from transfusion, ten IVDA). Only four patients had a complete response with complete normalization of ALT during therapy. After cessation of therapy, three relapsed, leaving only one patient with sustained normalization of ALT twelve months after the end of therapy. This patient had an asymptomatic HIV infection (CDC Clinical Stage II) with 1120 CD_4 cell count (mm^3) before therapy. Similarly, Dalton, et al.,[48] in New York, report one of five patients treated with the standard dose of alfa-interferon realizing a sustained normalization of ALT six months after completing therapy. Levels of HCV-RNA were not reported in either of the prior studies.

A study of 14 asymptomatic HIV (CDC stage II), HCV infected patients treated with a one year high dose tapering regimen of alfa-interferon starting at nine MU daily and ending at three MU thrice weekly showed results similar to non-HIV patients.[49] Four patients showed sustained normalization of ALT values and undetectable HCV-RNA six months after treatment.

All of the patients in the latter study had CD_4 cell count of >200 mm^3 and three of the four patients with sustained normalization of ALT had CD_4 cell counts of >400 mm^3.

The current data concerning alfa-interferon treatment of HCV in HIV patients allows for only preliminary directions in treatment. Success appears to be limited to those patients with asymptomatic HIV infection with CD_4 cell counts >200 mm^3 and preferably >400 mm^3. Alfa-interferon receptors diminish in advanced HIV disease (i. e. CD_4 < 200mm^3) making response to alfa-interferon treatment less likely.[49]

In summary, the presence of HIV infection seems to worsen hepatitis C in some patients. The incidence of rapidly progressive liver disease is uncertain but clearly occurs in a minority. HCV viremia probably increases after onset of HIV infection. It is not known in cases with a sustained normalization of ALT after alfa-interferon treatment whether this will actually result in an increased life expectancy since HIV infection persists. Whether HCV has a deleterious effect on HIV disease is unknown.

References

1. Seeff LB, Zimmerman HJ, Wright EC, et al. A randomized, double-blind controlled trial of the efficacy of immune serum globulin for the prevention of post-transfusion hepatitis. *Gastroenterology* 1977; 72:111–121.

2. Seeff LB. Diagnosis, therapy, and prognosis of viral hepatitis. In: Zakin D, Boyer TD, eds. *Hepatology: a textbook of liver disease.* Philadelphia: WB Saunders, 1990.

3. Sanchez-Quijara A, Pineda JA, Lissen E, et al. Prevention of post-transfusion non-A, non-B hepatitis by non-specific immunoglobulin in heart surgery patients. *Lancet* 1988; 1:1245–1249.

4. Kuhns WJ, Prince AM, Brotman B, et al. A clinical and laboratory evluation of immune serum globulin from donors with a history of

hepatitis: attempted prevention of post-transfusion hepatitis. *Am J Med Sci* 1976; 272:255–261.

5. Knodell RG, Conrad ME, Ginsberg AL, et al. Efficacy of prophylactic gamma-globulin in preventing non-A, non-B post-transfusion hepatitis. *Lancet* 1976: 1:557–561.

6. Kikuchi K, Tuteda A. The venoglobulin research group. *J Jpn Soc Blood Transfus* 1980; 24:2 (note: the author has been unable to obtain a copy of this article).

7. Conrad ME, Lemon SM. Prevention of endemic icteric viral hepatitis by administration of immune serum gamma globulin. *J Infect Dis* 1987; 156:56–63.

8. Farci P, Alter HJ, Wong D, et al. Attempts to neutralize hepatitis C virus *in vitro* with plasma from a chronically infected patient: evaluation in chimpanzees. *Hepatology* 1992; 16:105A (abstract).

9. Farci P, Alter HJ, Govindarajan S, et al. Lack of protective immunity against reinfection with hepatitis C virus. *Science* 1992; 258:135–139.

10. Lai ME, Mazzoleni AP, Argiolu F, et al. Hepatitis C virus in multiple episodes of acute hepatitis in poly transferred thalassaemic children. *Lancet* 1994; 343:388–389.

11. Miller MA, Orenstein P, Aminod B. Administration of immune serum globulin following exposure to hepatitis C virus. *Clin Infect Dis* 1993; 16:335.

12. Centers for Disease Control. *Protection against viral hepatitis.* Feb 9, 1990; 39:S-2.

13. Blanchette VS, Vorstman E, Shore A, et al. Hepatitis C infection in children with hemophilia A and B. *Blood* 1991; 78:285–289.

14. Locascialli A, Gornati G, Tagger A, et al. Hepatitis C virus infection and chronic liver disease in children with leukemia in long-term remission. *Blood* 1991; 78:1619–1622.

15. Jonas MM, Zilleruelo GE, LaRue SI, et al. Hepatitis C infection in a pediatric dialysis population. *Pediatrics* 1992; 89:707–709.

16. Maggiore G, De Giacoma C. Chronic viral hepatitis in children. *Arch Virol Suppl* 1992; 4:259–262.

17. Bortolotti F, Vajro P, Cadrobbi P, et al. Cryptogenic chronic liver disease and hepatitis C virus infection in children. *J Hepatology* 1992; 15:73–76.

18. Thaler MM, Fang H, Heyman MB. Giant cell hepatitis due to hepatitis C. *Hepatology* 1992; 16:74A (abstract).

19. Resti M, Azzari C, Rossi ME, et al. Hepatitis C virus antibodies in long-term follow-up of beta-thalassaemic children with acute and chronic non-A non-B hepatitis. *Eur J Ped* 1992; 151:573–576.

20. Di Marco V, Lo Iacono O, Capra M, et al. Alpha-interferon treatment of chronic hepatitis C in young patients with homozygous beta-thalassemia. *Haematologica* 1992; 77:502–506.

21. Ruiz-Moreno M, Rua MJ, Castillo I, et al. Treatment of children with chronic hepatitis C with recombinant interferon alpha: a pilot study. *Hepatology* 1992; 16:882–885.

22. Hieber JP, Dalton D, Shorey J. Hepatitis and pregnancy. *J Peds* 1977; 91:545–549.

23. Bohman VR, Stettler RW, Little BB, et al. Seroprevalence and risk factors for hepatitis C virus antibody in pregnant women. *Obstet Gynecol* 1992; 80:609–613.

24. Lee WM. Pregnancy in patients with chronic liver disease. *Gastroenterology Clinics N Amer* 1992; 21:889–903.

25. Ogasawara S, Kage M, Kosai KI. Hepatitis C virus RNA in saliva and breast milk of hepatitis C carrier mothers. *Lancet* 1993; 341:561.

26. Hsu H, Wright TL, Luba D, et al. Is hepatitis C virus in human secretions? *Gastenterology* 1991; 100:754 (abstract).

27. Johnson RJ, Gretch DR, Yamabe H, et al. Membranoproliferative glomerulonephritis associated with hepatitis C infection. *N Engl J Med* 1993; 328:465–470.

28. Davda R, Peterson J, Weiner R, et al. Membranous glomerulonephritis in association with hepatitis C virus infection. *Am J Kid Dis* 1993; 22:452–455.

29. Rostoker G, Deforges L, Ben Maadi A, et al. Low prevalence of hepatitis C virus antibodies among adult patients with primary gloerulonephritis in France. *Nephron* 1993; 63:367.

30. Holzberger G, Seidl S, Peschke B, et al. Second generation anti-HCV test: seroprevalence in hemodialysis and blood donors. *Transplant Proceedings* 1992; 24:2648–649.

31. Getzug T, Brezina M, Lindsay K, et al. Hepatitis C virus antibody in hemodialysis patients: comparison of prevalence using first and second generation assays. *Hepatology* 1990; 12:845 (abstract).

32. Chan TM, Lok AS, Cheng IK, et al. A prospective study of hepatitis C virus infection among renal transplant recipients. *Gastroenterology* 1993; 104:862–868.

33. Neves PL, Amorim JP. Should patients with hpeatitis C virus antibodies in chronic hemodialysis be isolated? *Am J Kid Dis* 1992; 20:422.

34. De Marchi S, Cecchin E, Villalta D, et al. Relief of pruritus and decreases in plasma histamine concentrations during erythropoietin therapy in patients with uremia. *N Engl J Med* 1992; 326:969–94.

35. Di Benedetto A, Biolatta E, Minale S, et al. Anti-HCV antibody presence in hemodialyzed patients: assessment after one year regarding some preventative measures chosen. *Nephron* 1992; 61:356–357.

36. Pol S, Legendre C, Saltiel C, et al. Hepatitis C virus in kidney recipients. *J Hepat* 1992; 15:202–206.

37. Ynares C, Johnson HK, Kerlin T, et al. Impact of pretransplant hepatitis C antibody status upon long-term patient and renal allograft survival—a 5 and 10 year follow-up. *Transplant Proc* 1993; 25:1466–468.

38. Morales JM, Munoz MA, Castellano G, et al. Impact of hepatitis C in long-functioning renal transplants: a clinicopathological follow-up. *Trans Proc* 1993; 25:1450–1453.

39. Eyster ME, Diamondstone LS, Lien JM, et al. Natural history of hepatitis C virus infection in multitransfused hemophiliacs: effect of coinfection with human immunodeficiency virus. *J AIDS* 1993; 6:602–610.

40. Martin P, Di Bisceglie AM, Kasaianides C, et al. Rapidly progressive non-A, non-B hepatitis in patients with human immunodeficiency virus infection. *Gastroenterology* 1989; 97:1559–1561.

41. Watson HG, Zhang LQ, Simmonds P, et al. Hepatitis C virus load increases with time after HIV infection. *Int Conf AIDS 1992* July 19-24; B195 [abstract no PoB 3629).

42. McNair AN, Main J, Thomas HC. Interactions of the human immunodeficiency virus and the hpeatotropic viruses. *Sem Liver Dis* 1992; 12:188–196.

43. Eyster ME, Fried MW, Di Bisceglie AM, et al. HCV-RNA in hemophiliacs with antibody to hepatitis C virus: relationship to HIV infection and liver failure. *Int AIDS Conference, Berlin, 1993* [abstract]. Courtesy, ME Eyster.

44. Areias J, Lopes I. Influence of HIV infection in chronic hepatitis C in intravenous drug addicts. *Hepatology* 1992; 16:195 (abstract).

45. Wright TL, Hollander H, Kim M. Hepatitis C viremia in human immunodeficiency virus infected patients with and without AIDS. *Hepatology* 1992; 16:70 (abstract).

46. Eyster ME, Alter HJ, Aledort LM. Heterosexual co-transmission of hepatitis C virus and human immunodeficiency virus. *Ann Intern Med* 1991; 115:764–768.

47. Boyer N, Marcellin P, Degott C, et al. Recombinant interferon-α for chronic hepatitis C in patients positive for antibody to human immunodeficiency virus. *J Infect Dis* 1992; 165:723–726.

48. Dalton, BH, Acosta A, Jacobson IM. Interferon therapy in HIV-positive patients with chronic hepatitis C. *Hepatology* 1992; 16:199 (abstract).
49. Marriott E, Nauns S, del Romero J, et al. Treatment with recombinant α-interferon on chronic hepatitis C in anti-HIV positive patients. *J Med Virology* 1993; 40:107–111.

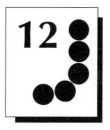

Treatment of Hepatitis C

Treatment with Alfa-Interferon 2b
Liver Transplantation

A cute hepatitic C leads to a chronic carrier state in the majority of those infected. A significant proportion of patients, ranging from 20% or more, may develop cirrhosis over several decades. A few patients can develop liver failure one to five years after infection. Chronic hepatitis C carriers with cirrhosis are at risk of developing hepatocellular carcinoma (Chapter 10).

A large seroprevalence study by the CDC shows 1.8% or 4.5 million people in the United States to be chronically infected with hepatitis C (unpublished). While disease due to hepatitis C is aggressive in a minority of carriers, HCV is so prevalent that it has become the most common indication for liver transplantation in the United States.

The approval of alfa-interferon 2b for use in chronic hepatitis C by the United States Food and Drug Administration in 1991 represents a milestone in the field of viral hepatitis. Alfa-interferon 2b is the first effective therapy for both chronic hepatitis B and C.

In contrast with hepatitis B, workers in hepatitis C are careful to use the terms "response" and "remission" rather than "disappearance" or

Table 12.1 Nomenclature.

ALT—alanine aminotransferase (formerly SGPT)

AST—aspartate aminotransferase (formerly SGOT)

MU—million units

Complete response—reduction of ALT into the normal range

Partial response—reduction of ALT but values are still above normal

Non-response—no change in ALT values

Sustained response—ALT values remain normal for 6 to 24 months after cessation of interferon therapy

Relapse—ALT values return to pre-treatment values

Alpha-interferon—naturally derived from mammalian sources

Alfa-interferon—recombinant produced human interferon

"cure" since current technology does not allow direct identification of the hepatitis C virus. A method called the polymerase chain reaction (Chapter 9) is being used in research studies to monitor HCV-RNA levels as a measure of viral replication in serum during and after treatment.[1–3] Assays for HCV-RNA in serum and liver may provide a more direct way to monitor treatment responses, but these methods are cumbersome, expensive and lack reproducibility. For practical treatment, surrogate markers, such as the aminotransferases ALT and AST, are employed to monitor inflammation and viral replication during treatment. A complete response to alfa-interferon occurs when ALT values fall into the normal range. A sustained response takes place when ALT values remain normal for more than six months after therapy. Table 12.1 outlines the nomenclature of therapy.

A rough correlation exists between HCV-RNA levels and the elevation of the ALT value, but disparity can occur.[4] Loss of HCV-RNA in the serum or liver at the end of treatment does not necessarily predict a sustained remission.[5]

However, continued disappearance of serum HCV-RNA six months after therapy appears to correlate well with long-term absence of the virus.[6]

Treatment of Hepatitis C with Alfa-Interferon

Interferons are a class of proteins produced by mammalian cells with a wide spectrum of antiviral, antiproliferative and immunomodulatory effects (Table 12.2).[7] Monocytes and lymphocytes make alfa-interfer-

Table 12.2 The actions of interferons. Derived from M. Peters. Mechanisms of actions of interferons. *Sem Liver Dis* 1989; 9:235–9.

Decrease

— Viral entry

— Viral mRNA synthesis

— Viral protein synthesis

Activate

— Macrophages

— Cytotoxic T-cells

— Natural killer cells

Increase

— Cell membrane proteins

— 2'5' oligo-adenylate synthetase

ons in response to viral and antigenic stimuli. After cellular uptake, interferons induce proteins that mediate antiviral actions. A virus, by definition, cannot synthesize proteins or nucleic acids. It must take over the cellular mechanisms of the host cell to replicate (Figure 12.1). Alfa-interferon stimulates a protein called 2'5'-oligo-adenylate synthetase that appears to inhibit takeover of cell synthesis by the virus.[7]

Invasion of a host cell by a virus results in expression of proteins onto the cell surface. Inhibition of these signals must occur for a virus to escape recognition by circulating lymphocytes and establish a chronic presence. Alfa-interferon appears to promote the surface expression of membrane proteins; these *marked* cells can then be destroyed by cytotoxic T-cells.[7]

The reasons why some patients respond to alfa-interferon and others do not are poorly understood.

Alfa-interferon was first reported effective for the treatment of chronic non-A, non-B hepatitis in 1986.[8] Ten patients with well-characterized non-A, non-B hepatitis were treated with recombinant human alpha-interferon. Subcutaneous injections of two to five million units (MU) were administered three times each week. Eight patients showed a sustained reduction in aminotransferase levels for twelve months. Liver biopsies documented improvement in portal inflammation and hepatocyte necrosis. Subsequent randomized, controlled trials have proven the effectiveness of alfa-interferon treatment (at a dose of 3 MU

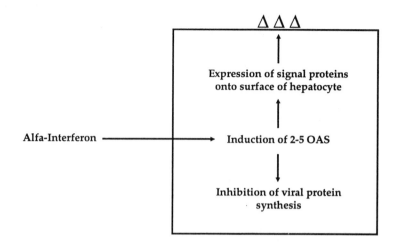

Figure 12.1 Diagram of anti-viral events caused by alfa-interferon in a hepatocyte. 2-5OAS = 2′5′-oligo-adenylate synthetase.

thrice weekly for six months) for chronic HCV infection.[9,10] Up to a point, the probability of response is both time dependent and dose related. A recent meta-analysis of randomized controlled interferon trials reveals 50% of patients normalize their aminotransferases while on treatment.[10] Responders to interferon also improve histologically.[11,12] However, 50% of responding patients relapse after treatment, leaving only 20–25% of patients with a sustained response after treatment.[10]

No clinical, demographic, biochemical, serological or histologic characteristics have been identified that reliably predict patients response.[13,14] Some studies have found younger age, lack of cirrhosis and low viremia levels (i.e., HCV-RNA) to be predictors of a positive response.[15–17] In a small study of six patients, increasing amino acid heterogeneity in the variable regions of the E2/NSI viral protein has been found in non-responsive patients. This suggests a variable population of hepatitis C virus quasispecies occurs in non-responders to interferon. A significant change in the hepatitis C virus quasispecies population takes place in patients after interferon treatment, possibly reflecting a differential sensitivity to interferon, selective immune pressure by the host or both.[18]

Side-effects

Alfa-interferon can cause undesirable reactions. A review of the U.S. multicenter trial (Figure 12.2) shows responses different from placebo.[9]

Fever, myalgia and headache can occur for 4–12 hours after the first injection or two but this reaction usually subsides or disappears by the third or fourth injection. These initial symptoms are ameliorated by taking acetaminophen one hour after the injection and every four hours as necessary. Some patients also find diphenhydramine helpful, particularly at night. For management of symptomatic side-effects of alfa-interferon, please refer to Table 8.5.

Many patients complain of fatigue during therapy; but in the U. S. trial, those patients reporting this symptom did not differ in number from placebo. Fatigue may be a manifestation of HCV rather than treatment. Regardless, it is rare for patients to miss a work day due to this symptom while taking alfa-interferon.

Depression and irritability were no more common among treated patients than those receiving placebo in the U.S. trial. Nonetheless, others report 10% of patients can suffer psychiatric symptoms with depression most common.[19] Three patients (out of fifty treated) developed major depression episodes during treatment requiring reduction of dose and psychiatric treatment (personal observation). All three

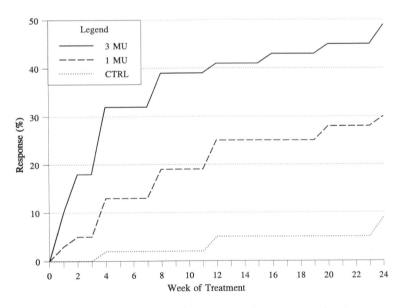

Figure 12.2 Probability of complete or near-complete response during treatment with recombinant interferon alfa in patients with chronic hepatitis C (3 MU denotes a dose of 3 million units of interferon thrice weekly, 1 MU a dose of 1 million units thrice weekly and CTRL untreated. Reprinted, by permission of the *New England Journal of Medicine*, vol. 321; page 1504, 1989.

patients had a history of psychiatric problems before treatment. A history of psychiatric problems is a relative contraindication to alfa-interferon therapy. If therapy is elected, it is wise to have such a patient see a psychiatrist regularly during therapy. Regardless of past psychiatric history, all patients and spouses should be counseled about the possibility of irritability and depression occurring during treatment.

Mild alopecia and diarrhea can occur and will resolve after cessation of therapy. A few patients may have an acceleration of their male pattern of baldness.[19]

The development of autoantibodies, with or without autoimmune disease, occurs in more than 50% of patients treated with alfa-interferon. Fortunately, overt autoimmune disease is rare; the most common manifestation is autoimmune thyroiditis associated with either hypo- or hyperthyroidism.[19,20] In clinical trials, <1% (4/426) developed thyroid abnormalities.[21]

Alfa-interferon is mildly myelosuppressive. In the 3 MU thrice weekly dose, 15% of patients experience a hemoglobin decline of ≥ 2 gm/dl; 18% will have the white cell count decline to under 3,000 mm^3; and 9% will develop thrombocytopenia with a platelet count of less than 70,000/mm^3.[13] The mild myelosuppression is surprisingly well tolerated in those who start with normal hematologic values. Patients with cirrhosis and hypersplenism can have marked decreases in peripheral cell counts that may limit therapy. Decreasing the dose of alfa-interferon will ameliorate the reduction in blood counts to some extent. Reversal of myelosuppression occurs within a few weeks of stopping therapy.

Bacterial infections are the most serious side effect of therapy. Cases of septicemia, lung abscess, brain abscess and bacterial peritonitis are reported.[19] Cirrhotics, who already have significant humoral immunity defects, are particularly predisposed. Any fever occurring after the first two weeks of therapy deserves an immediate evaluation. The clinician should have a low threshold to start antibiotics.

Clinicians or patients considering alfa-interferon treatment for hepatitis C are cautioned against being overly concerned with the side-effects of alfa-interferon listed for cancer therapy. Many reactions occur only at very high doses (i.e. 10 to 20 million units daily) used in cancer treatment and do not take place at the low dose (3 million three times weekly) used for hepatitis C. While cardiovascular responses such as arrhythmias or heart failure may arise in high dose therapy, the U. S. trial for hepatitis C did not report cardiac complications. However, patients with significant cardiovascular disease were excluded by major trials and thus cardiovascular tolerance is not well tested. Fever with resultant tachycardia can aggravate angina pectoris or underlying arrhythmias. Patients with symptomatic cardiovascular disease are therefore poor candidates for alfa-interferon 2b therapy.

All patients will experience side effects to some degree. In large trials, a dose reduction took place in 15% and stopping therapy due to side effects occurred in 5%.[9,11,22] Physicians and patients should be aware of the possible side-effects of alfa-interferon and remain in communication. If the treating physician has not been trained in alfa-interferon use, it is recommended they thoroughly read the package insert.

Selection of patients for treatment

Since alfa-interferon is expensive, associated with side-effects (usually temporary), and has a 25% sustained remission rate after therapy, all patients with chronic hepatitis C are not candidates for therapy.

The National Institutes of Health (NIH) and the National Hepatitis Detection and Treatment Program have issued guidelines for those patients with chronic hepatitis C who are eligible for treatment with alfa-interferon (Tables 12.3 and 12.4).[23,24] At the core of these guidelines, patients are selected who appear to have *progressive liver disease* due to hepatitis C but who have not yet *decompensated* with complications from the disease. As reviewed in Chapter 10, 20% or more of patients with chronic HCV may progress to chronic liver disease and ultimately cirrhosis.

All clinicians agree that patients with progressive liver disease should be treated. In patients with minimal liver disease, treatment is more controversial. The trend is now to consider earlier use of alfa-interferon 2b. Reasons for considering therapy in patients with minimal liver disease include symptoms of fatigue, marked anxiety over the variable prognosis of hepatitic C and possibility of disease transmission. In the later group, the author considers young women who may become pregnant or health care workers as candidates for treatment.

Given the lack of serological markers that accurately predict progressive disease, the best understanding is obtained through a liver biopsy. The discovery of severe chronic active hepatitis, bridging necrosis or active cirrhosis establishes the presence of progressive liver disease. A liver biopsy also helps to exclude other causes of chronic liver disease such as hemochromatosis or alpha-one antitrypsin deficiency.

Liver biopsy is not necessary in the evaluation of all hepatitis C patients. The NIH recommends investigating patients who have biochemical evidence of severe disease as defined by persistently elevated aminotransferases (greater than 5–10 times the upper limit of the

Table 12.3 Side effects of interferon treatment in patients with chronic hepatitis C. Reprinted, by permission of the *New England Journal of Medicine*, volume 321; page 1504, 1989.

	Interferon Dose		
	None	**1 Million Units**	**3 Million Units**
No. of Patients	51	57	58
		number (percent)	
Any symptom	50 (98)	56 (98)	55 (95)
Fever	3 (6)	24 (42)*	28 (48)*
Myalgia	2 (4)	23 (40)*	32 (55)*
Headache	9 (18)	27 (47)†	31 (53)*
Diarrhea	4 (8)	13 (23)	20 (34)†
Alopecia	0 (0)	5 (9)	14 (24)*
Arthralgia	4 (8)	10 (18)	9 (16)
Rash	2 (4)	8 (14)	7 (12)
Injection-site erythema	0 (0)	4 (7)	5 (9)
Depression	4 (8)	5 (9)	8 (14)
Fatigue	39 (76)	44 (77)	45 (78)
Nausea	11 (22)	18 (32)	21 (36)
Irritability	12 (24)	17 (30)	16 (28)

*P<0.001 versus untreated group   †P<0.003 versus untreated group

Table 12.4 General guidelines for eligibility of patients with chronic HCV for alfa–interferon treatment.

- Presence of symptoms which interfere with daily life
- Persistently and markedly elevated ALT values (> 5×normal)
- Histological evidence of progressive liver disease
    - Chronic active hepatitis
    - Bridging necrosis
    - Active cirrhosis

normal range) or the presence of symptoms that interfere with daily life.[15]

The initial evaluation should uncover no other causes for chronic liver disease. Alcohol, drug, metabolic or autoimmune induced hepatitis must be considered. Autoimmune hepatitis is difficult to exclude since patients with this disease and hyperglobulinemia can test false-positive for anti-HCV. Unfortunately, secondary assays for HCV antigens, such as RIBA-II or HCV-RNA, do not accurately classify AIH patients.[25] Absence of significant antinuclear antibody levels and normal immunoglobulin levels help exclude AIH.[23] Ultimately, a short trial of therapy with corticosteroids may be necessary to determine whether the chronic active hepatitis is due to AIH (see Chapter 9).

Whether the chronic active hepatitis is due to HCV or AIH is critical since treatment with alfa-interferon worsens AIH.[26] On the other hand, treatment of HCV with corticosteroids probably causes no harm. Therefore, if the diagnosis of AIH is in doubt, a course of corticosteroids is indicated first rather than alfa-interferon.

For the non-liver specialist, patients being considered for therapy should not have clinical or laboratory evidence for decompensated liver disease. Hepatic encephalopathy, variceal bleeding, ascites or markedly abnormal laboratory values (Table 12.5) are parameters of the decompensated state. Patients with decompensated disease are more prone to have an adverse event such as bleeding or infection during therapy. In the author's experience, severe thrombocytopenia (<50,000 platelets/cm^3), is often a limiting factor in the treatment of advanced liver disease due to hepatitis C.

In addition to liver disease, associated medical problems may exclude the patient from alfa-interferon therapy. Interferon should be used cautiously in patients with debilitating medical conditions who may not safely tolerate side effects. These conditions include a history of uncontrolled diabetes mellitus, severe COPD, coagulation disorders, myelosuppression or HIV disease. Patients with a history of autoimmune disease should not be treated with interferon, since its immunomodulatory effects can worsen the disease.

Table 12.5 Pretreatment evaluation of chronic hepatitis C for alfa-interferon treatment.

- Serum ALT, bilirubin, albumin, creatinine
- Complete blood count, platelet count, prothrombin time
- Measurement of thyroid-stimulating hormone activity
- Liver biopsy
- Assessment of mental status

Alfa-interferon is approved for use only in patients over age 18.[21] Children with chronic HCV do not appear to be at risk of developing cirrhosis before adulthood (see Chapter 11).

Doses

A dose of three MU is superior to one MU.[11,27–28] With three million units three times a week, the response is 46%, contrasted with a 28% response rate in patients receiving one million units three times a week. Augmenting the dose to six MU in "non-responders" does not seem to induce a biochemical response.[28] The recommended dosage for alfa-interferon is three million IU three times a week, for 24 weeks, administered subcutaneously or intramuscularly. Normalization of aminotransferase levels can occur in some patients as early as two weeks after initiation of therapy. Patients who respond to alfa-interferon with a reduction in aminotransferase levels should complete 24 weeks of therapy. The manufacturer recommends evaluation of response after 16 weeks. Therapy should be stopped if aminotransferases remain elevated after 16 weeks of treatment.[21]

Increasing the dose of alfa-interferon to five to 7.5 MU does not appear to improve the rate of sustained remission. However, preliminary evidence is suggestive that longer duration of treatment may be helpful, particularly in those with significant fibrosis.[29] The optimal duration of therapy remains under investigation. Until further data is available, the standard dose of three MU given three times weekly for 24 weeks should be considered the optimal regimen since it achieves maximal results with minimal expense and side effects.

Monitoring

The goals of monitoring are to identify toxicity and response to treatment. A CBC and platelet count should be measured 2 weeks after therapy is started and monthly throughout treatment. TSH testing should be done at three and, if necessary, six months of treatment.[21] ALT is measured after two and 16 weeks of therapy. If the ALT is normal at 16 weeks, treatment is continued for eight more weeks and the ALT rechecked. After therapy is completed, measurement of the ALT can be done quarterly for the first year and semiannually for the second year following therapy.

The end point of therapeutic response is called a long-term remission and this is defined as a persistently normal ALT for two years after treatment is stopped. In this clinical context, HCV-RNA levels are usually undetectable.

Six of the ten patients first treated by the NIH have had a long-term remission of three to six years. ALT values are normal and HCV RNA levels undetectable. All six patients have no signs of parenchymal inflammation or of hepatitis C activity. Anti-HCV antibody levels, however, have declined only minimally.[35]

Four Italian patients in long-term remission underwent liver biopsy two years after end of therapy. All four patients had normal histology compared with chronic active hepatitis in three and chronic persistent hepatitis in one before therapy. Three of the four were negative for HCV-RNA.[36]

Relapse

Half of patients who completely respond to alfa-interferon will relapse with abnormal ALT values after therapy is discontinued. In some cases, a transient, self-limited relapse occurs followed by a long-term improvement.[14]

The NIH reported a second course of therapy for an additional year in two relapsers with recurrence of elevated ALT values after cessation of the second treatment.[35] Studies of ten patients in Sweden and 20 patients in Italy retreated show similar outcomes of disease recurrence.[37,38] The author also has had uniform relapses in patients treated a second time.

A large, multicenter five year trial (started in 1993) is in progress looking at titrating long-term doses of alfa-interferon for patients who have relapsed with standard therapy. Sustained treatment with alfa-interferon is not without difficulty. In the 60 week treatment study cited earlier, three out of 41 patients had major adverse effects. One patient had significant alopecia, another had hypothyroidism and the third patient developed polymyositis.[34]

Cost-effectiveness

The cost of six months of alfa-interferon is about $2,000 at our institution. While cost-benefit analyses are contrived to some degree, Figure 12.3 outlines the potential cost of therapy versus the cost of liver transplantation.

Figure 12.3 presents the direct charges for alfa-interferon versus direct charges for initial liver transplantation (median charge $172,000 in 1992[39]). Ongoing maintenance of a transplant ($10,000 per year) is not included. The point to be made about cost and benefit is that there is a log order (ten times) difference in cost versus benefit.

Others have published a cost-benefit analysis of alfa-interferon therapy with favorable conclusions.[40,41]

Transplantation for End-Stage Liver Disease Due to Hepatitis C

While hepatitis C (HCV) causes progressive liver disease and eventual liver failure in a minority of carriers, it is the most common indication for liver transplantation.[42,43] Unfortunately, receiving a new liver does not cure the infection. The detection of recurrent HCV in the post-transplant setting is underestimated with EIA or RIBA II testing.[44] With HCV-RNA testing, 93% of patients transplanted for liver disease due to HCV develop recurrent infection in the new liver with HCV.[45] In contrast to hepatitis B, many patients with recurrent HCV have very mild, if any, disease and seldom develop liver failure. A series of 58 patients from San Francisco transplanted for HCV with a median follow-up of 25 months showed two patients who died from liver failure, two re-transplanted for recurrent HCV disease and one alive with cirrhosis.[45] An Italian series shows similar results.[44] Thus, significant disease development at two years appears to be around 10%.

Transplantation of the liver for end-stage liver disease caused by HCV is a valid and acceptable therapy. Eligibility for transplantation, then, depends on associated diseases and other factors rather than on the presence or absence of HCV.

Summary

No outline of alfa-interferon 2b treatment of chronic hepatitis C is provided at the end of this chapter. Physicians wishing to use this therapy should thoroughly read this chapter and the product insert to familiarize themselves with alfa-interferon. Tables 12.4–12.6 outline pretreatment evaluation and eligibility.

Table 12.6 Laboratory guidelines for eligibility. Derived from Intron® A. *Physicians Desk Reference.* Medical Economicx Data. Montrale, NJ. 1994.

Bilirubin ≤ 2mg/dl

Albumin—within normal limits

Prothrombin time < 3 seconds prolonged

WBC ≥ 3,000/mm³

Platelets ≥ 70,000/mm³

Serum creatinine at or near normal

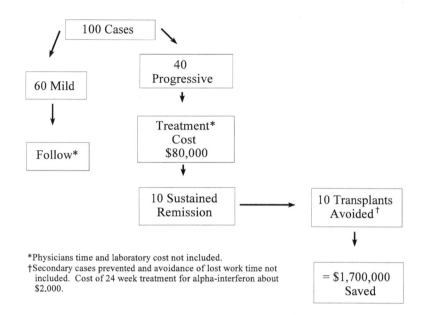

Figure 12.3 Cost analysis of treating progressive liver disease due to chronic hepatitis C.

References

1. Schlauder G, Leverenz G, Mattsson L, et al. Detection of hepatitis C viral RNA by the polymerase chain reaction in serum of patients with post-transfusion non-A, non-B hepatitis. *J Virol Methods*, 1992; 37:189–199.

2. Brillanti S, Garson J, Tuke P, et al. Effect of alfa-interferon therapy on hepatitis C viraemia in community-acquired chronic non-A, non-B hepatitis: A quantitative polymerase chain reaction study. *J Med Virol* 1991; 34:136–141.

3. Chayama K, Saitoh S, Arase Y, et al. Effect of interferon administration of serum hepatitis C virus RNA in patients with chronic hepatitis C. *Hepatology* 1991; 13:1040–1043.

4. Kurosaki M, Enomoto N, Sato C, et al. Correlation of plasma hepatitis C virus RNA levels with serum alanine aminotransferase in non-A, non-B chronic liver disease. *J Med Virology* 1993; 39:246–250.

5. Balart LA, Perrillo R, Roddenberry J, et al. Hepatitis C RNA in liver of chronic hepatitis C patients before and after interferon alfa treatment. *Gastroenterology* 1993; 104:1472–1477.

6. Morisco F, Tuccillo C, S, Sessa G, et al. Can chronic HCV infection terminate in patients with chronic active hepatitis long-term re-

sponders to interferon therapy? *Gastroenterology* 1995; 108:1126 (abstract).

7. Peters M. Mechanisms of actions of interferons. *Sem Liver Dis* 1989; 9:235–239.

8. Hoofnagle JH, Mullen KD, Jones D, et al. Treatment of chronic non-A, non-B hepatitis with recombinant human alpha interferon. A preliminary report. *N Engl J Med* 1986; 315:1575–1578.

9. Davis G, Balart L, Schiff E, et al. Treatment of chronic hepatitis C with recombinant interferon alfa. A multicenter randomized, controlled trial. *N Engl J Med* 1989; 321:1501–1506.

10. Tine F, Magrin S, Craxi A, et al. Interferon for non-A, non-B chronic hepatitis. A meta-analysis of randomized clinical trials. *J Hepatol* 1991; 13:192–199.

11. Di Bisceglie A, Martin P, Kassianides C, et al. Recombinant interferon alfa therapy for chronic hepatitis C. A randomized, double-blind controlled trial. *N Engl J Med* 1989; 321:1506–1510.

12. Schvarez R, Glaumann H, Weiland O, et al. Histological outcome in interferon alpha-2b treated patients with chronic post-transfusion non-A non-B hepatitis. *Liver* 1991; 11:30–38.

13. Davis G, Lindsay K, Albrecht J, et al. Predictors of response to recombinant alpha interferon (rIFN) treatment in patients with chronic hepatitis C. *Hepatology* 1990; 12:905 (abstract).

14. Lindsay K, Davis G, Bodenheimer H, et al. Predictors of relapse and response to re-treatment in patients with an initial response to recombinant alpha interferon therapy for chronic hepatitis C. *Hepatology* 1990; 12:847.

15. Rubin RA, Falestiny M, Malet PF. Chronic hepatitis C: advances in diagnostic testing and therapy. *Arch Intern Med* 1994; 154:387–392.

16. Camps J, Crisostomo S, Garcia-Granero M, et al. Predication of the response of chronic hepatitis C to interferon alfa: a statistical analysis of pretreatment variables. *Gut* 1993; 34:1714–1717.

17. Jouet P, Roudot-Thoraval F, Dhumeaux D, et al. Comparative efficacy of interferon alfa in cirrhotic and noncirrhotic patients with non-A, non-B, C hepatitis. *Gastroenterology* 1994; 106:686–690.

18. Okada S, Akahane Y, Suzuki H, et al. The degree of variability in the amino terminal region of the E2/NS1 protein of hepatitis C virus correlates with responsiveness to interferon therapy in viremic patients. *Hepatology* 1992; 16:619–624.

19. Renault PF, Hoofnagle JH. Side affects of alpha interferon. *Sem Liver Dis* 1989; 9:273–277.

20. Marcellin P, Pouteau M, Renard P, et al. Sustained hypothyroidism induced by recombinant α-interferon in patients with chronic hepatitis C. *Gut* 1992; 33:855–856.

21. Intron® A. *Physicians Desk Reference*. Medical Economics Data. Montvale, NJ. 1995.

22. Jacyna M, Brooks M, Loke RH, et al. Randomized controlled trial of interferon alpha (lymphoblastoid interferon) in chronic non-A non-B hepatitis. *BMJ* 1989; 298:80–82.

23. Di Bisceglie AM, Hoofnagle JH. Therapy of chronic hepatitis C with α-interferon: the answer? or more questions? *Hepatology* 1991; 13:601–603.

24. Experts achieve consensus on hepatitis C therapy. *Issues in Hepatitis* 1992; 2:1-4 (published by Advanced Therapeutic Communications, Secaucus, NJ 07094)

25. Nishiguchi S, Kuroki T, Ueda T, et al. Detection of hepatitis C virus antibody in the absence of viral RNA in patients with autoimmune hepatitis. *Ann Intern Med* 1992; 116:21–26.

26. Papo T, Marcellin P, Bernuau J, et al. Autoimmune chronic hepatitis exacerbated by alpha-interferon. *Ann Intern Med* 1992; 116:51–53.

27. Schvarcz T, Weiland O, Wejstal R, et al. A randomized controlled open study of interferon alpha-2b treatment of chronic non-A, non-B post-transfusion hepatitis: no correlation of outcome to presence of hepatitis C virus antibodies. *Scan J Infect Dis* 1989; 21:617–625.

28. Schvarcz R, Glaumann H, Weiland O, et al. Interferon alpha-2b treatment of chronic post-transfusion non-A, non-B/C hepatitis: long term outcome and effect of increased interferon doses in non-responders. *Scand J Infect Dis* 1991; 23:413–420.

29. Poynard T, Bedossa P, Chevalier M, et al. A comparison of three interferion alfa-2b regimens for long-term treatment of chronic non-A, non-B hepatitis. *N Engl J Med* 1995; 332:1457–62.

30. Colombo M, Rumi MG, Marcelli R, et al. Randomized controlled trial of recombinant alfa in patients with chronic hepatitis C. *Hepatology* 1991; 14:73 (abstract).

31. Metreau JM, Calmus Y, Poupon R, et al. Twelve-month treatment, compared to 6-month treatment, does not improve the efficacy of alpha-interferon in NANB chronic active hepatitis. *Hepatology* 1991; 14:72 (abstract).

32. Saez-Royuela F, Porres JC, Morero A, et al. High doses of recombinant α-interferon or gamma interferon for chronic hepatitis C: a randomized controlled trial. *Hepatology* 1991; 13:327–331.

33. Ferenci P, Vogel W, Hentschel E, et al. One year interferon alpha treatment of chronic hepatitis NANB. *Hepatology* 1991; 14:72 (abstract).

34. Reichard O, Foberg U, Fryden A, et al. High sustained response rate and clearance of viremia in chronic hepatitis C after treatment with interferon-alfa 2b for 60 weeks. *Hepatology* 1994; 19:280–285.

35. Shindo M, DiBisceglie, Hoofnagle JH. Long-term followup of patients with chronic hepatitis C treated with α-interferon. *Hepatology* 1992; 15:1013–1016.

36. Saracco G, Rosina F, Abate ML, et al. Long-term follow-up of patients with chronic hepatitis C treated with different doses of interferon-alfa 2b. *Hepatology* 1993; 18:1300–1305.

37. Weiland O, Zhang YY, Widell A. Serum HCV-RNA levels in patients with chronic hepatitis C given a second course of interferon alpha-2b treatment after relapse following initial treatment. *Scand J Infect Dis* 1993; 25:25–30.

38. Taliani G, Furlan C, Grimaldi F, et al. One course versus two course of recombinant alpha interferon in chronic C hepatitis. *Arch Virol Suppl* 1992; 4:294–298.

39. Organ procurement costs highest for liver, study finds. *Progress 1993*; 14:4 (published by the American Liver Foundation, Cedar Grove, NJ 07009).

40. Davis, GL. Recombinant α-interferon treatment of non-A, non-B (type C) hepatitis: review of studies and recommendations for treatment. *J Hepatology* 1990; 11:S72–77.

41. De Ancos JL, Roberts JA, Dusheiko GM. An economic evaluation of the costs of α-interferon treatment of chronic active hepatitis due to hepatitis B or C virus. *J Hepatology* 1990; S11–S18.

42. Belli LS, Alberti A, Rodinara GF, et al. Recurrent hepatitis C after liver transplantation. *Transplantation Proceedings* 1993; 25:2635–2637.

43. Shah G, Demetris AJ, Gavaler JS, et al. Incidence, prevalence and clinical course of hepatitis C following liver transplantation. *Gastroenterology* 1992; 103:323–329.

44. Wright TL. Liver transplantation for chronic hepatitis C viral infection. *Gastroenterology Clinics of North American* 1993; 22:231–242.

45. Lake JR, Wright T, Ferrell L, et al. Hepatitis C and B in liver transplantation. *Transplantation Proceedings* 1993; 25:2006–2009.

13

Delta Hepatitis

Discovery

In the mid 1970's Mario Rizzetto, a young gastroenterologist in Turin, Italy, discovered a "new" antigen by immunofluorescence microscopy in liver biopsy specimens from Italian patients with chronic hepatitis B. The particle was found to be antigenically distinct from hepatitis B core antigen. The peculiar antigen was never found in hepatitis B surface antigen (HBsAg) negative hepatitis and only in a proportion of patients who were HBsAg positive. The new marker was named delta antigen and its antibody anti-delta in the first report published in 1977.

Rizzetto pursued further investigations of delta antigen during a fellowship from the National Institutes of Health in the United States and with chimpanzee studies showed that the delta antigen was an internal component of a transmissible agent that required coinfection with hepatitis B for viral replication.[1]

Molecular studies led to the identification of a small (1700 nucleotides), single stranded RNA virus not resembling any known transmissible agent of animals; the delta virion resembles partial or subviral agents from the plant world which require the helper function of another virus.[2]

The delta subvirus (HDV) genome is so small that only one protein, hepatitis delta antigen (HDAg), is encoded. HDAg appears to form a complex with the HDV RNA genome. Hepatitis B surface antigen surrounds the inner delta complex completely to form a surface coat (Figure 13.1).[3, 4] As Purcell writes:

> Rizzetto's contributions in discovering HDV have been among the most significant and far reaching in the study of the basic science of the hepatitis viruses. Like Blumberg before him who made a chance discovery that might easily have been discarded, Rizzetto pursued a paradox until he understood it.[1]

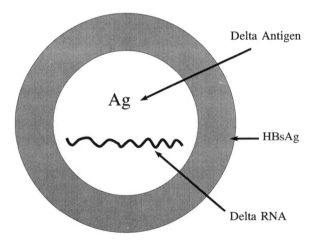

Figure 13.1 Structures of a delta virus. Delta antigen and RNA are complexed inside a coat of hepatitis B surface antigen.[3]

Clinical Features

Since HDV infection requires the presence of HBV as HBsAg, two modes of clinical expression are possible; one, HBV and HDV can be acquired at the same time as *coinfection*; secondly, HDV infection can be imposed on a chronic carrier of HBV as *superinfection* (Table 13.1). The clinical expression, incidence of fulminant hepatitis and chronic carrier rate differ between *coinfection* and *superinfection*.

In coinfection, HBsAg and HDAg appear in the serum several weeks apart, causing two peaks of aminotransferases (ALT) known as a *biphasic* or relapsing illness (Table 13.1). Biphasic illness has been reported in as few as 14% to as many as 80% of acute HDV co-infections.[5, 6] The first ALT peak denotes the immune response to HBsAg and the second peak to HDAg.

Superinfection of an HBV carrier causes acute hepatitis in 50–70% of patients. Asymptomatic infection can occur since 5% of HBsAg carriers with HDV antibodies have no prior history of hepatitis.[6]

In Milan, Italy, the clinical course of coinfection and superinfection were compared with acute uncomplicated hepatitis B. The diseases did not differ in average height of serum aminotransferase activities, bilirubin or prothrombin time; however, delta superinfection was a more severe disease as reflected by increased hospital time, prolonged illness and frequency of markedly elevated prothrombin time.[7] The diseases also differ in chronic carrier outcomes and incidence of fulminant hepatitis.

Coinfection seldom leads to a chronic carrier state of either HBV or HDV. The development of chronic carriers in this situation is reported to occur in 2.4–4.7% of cases. In contrast, superinfection with HDV leads to a chronic carrier state more than 90% of the time.[6, 7] The chronic carrier rate for young adults infected with acute hepatitis B alone is often cited at 5% but this rate differs markedly according to age and immunocompetence as noted in Chapter 4.

Table 13.1 Two modes of HDV acquisition. See text for differences in disease outcome.

Since delta virus requires the presence of hepatitis B virus, two modes of acquisition occur:	
Co-infection	*Superinfection*
HDV and HBV acquired simultaneously	HDV virus acquired by a chronic HBV carrier

The incidence of fulminant hepatitis as a result of the two acquisition modes of HDV seems to vary greatly in different parts of the world. In the tropical belt where there is a high rate of HBV endemicity, the majority of fulminant hepatitides associated with HDV occur in superinfection. In Western areas, outbreaks of fulminant HDV occur predominantly in drug addicts who acquire the infection simultaneously.[6,8]

Fulminant viral hepatitis is a rare sequelae of any type of acute viral hepatitis but is approximately ten times more common in delta hepatitis than in any other type of viral hepatitis.[9]

The mortality rate of acute delta hepatitis is 5% versus 1% for acute hepatitis B alone.[7] However, the mortality on short term follow-up of 126 cases of HDV in Los Angeles was 23% with 60% of deaths due to fulminant hepatitis.[10]

Extrahepatic disease

While HDV can replicate in non-liver cells *in vitro*, extrahepatic disease in patients with HDV has not been documented. Several case reports describe Guillain-Barré syndrome or other neurologic difficulties[6;] it seems probable that these are complications from HBV since neurologic deficits are well-described for HBV (Chapter 4).

Hepatocellular carcinoma

Delta infection does *not* confer an increased incidence of hepatocellular carcinoma (HCC).[6,11] When delta antibody is found in patients with HCC, the lack of HDAg and IgM antibody indicate that the antibody is a marker of resolved infection.[11]

The reason for this non-association of HCC and HDV may be ominous; the liver disease caused by HDV is much more rapidly progressive than in HBV (see natural history section) so that affected patients may die before they have a chance to develop HCC.

Diagnosis

The only commercially available assay for diagnosis of HDV infection in the United States is a blocking RIA test for total antibody (anti-HD) to delta antigen. Anti-HD measures both IgG and IgM antibodies, though in practice, the principal antibody is IgG.[8] The problem with anti-HD is the inability to detect acute delta coinfection or superinfection at the onset of symptoms. In one study of acute coinfection, 15%

of cases were positive at admission while in 92% it was found after 30 days.[12]

Delta antigen (HDAg), IgM antibody to HDAg (IgM anti-HD) and HDV-RNA assays are available overseas and only on a research basis in the United States. HDAg occurs in low titer and is short-lived (less than a week) in acute infection.[7] Only 35% of patients with acute delta infection have this marker upon admission.[12] IgM anti-HD can also appear late and last briefly. 31% of acute infections initially have IgM antibody present.[12] It lasts for about two weeks and disappears in resolving infections after 21 to 43 days.[13]

Little information is available on HDV-RNA. If all markers of HDV are utilized, only 69% of patients can be correctly diagnosed at the onset of illness. Thus, the most cost effective approach of testing for *acute* HDV infection during an acute illness of HBV is to measure total anti-HD 30 to 40 days after the onset of symptoms.[12] *Chronic* delta infection is simple to diagnose since anti-HD levels will be persistently high.

If acute infection resolves, anti-HD levels will disappear in one to two years. The finding of anti-HD in a carrier of HBsAg is therefore much more likely to reflect underlying infection than past exposure to HDV.[8]

Epidemiology and Transmission

Since HDV is dependent upon HBV, the epidemiology of HDV infection is similar to HBV but with notable exceptions. Worldwide, there are about 300 million HBsAg carriers and it is estimated that at least 5% of these carriers also have delta infection.[14]

North America is considered a low endemic area for HDV. Delta antibodies have been found in 1% (south-central) to 12% (San Jose, California) of HBsAg positive blood donors in the United States.[15] 4% of acute hepatitis B is attributable to HDV and 2% of all acute viral hepatitis in the U. S. is thought secondary to HDV.[16] The prevalence is highest in those chronic HBV groups (Figure 13.4) with repeated percutaneous exposure such as intravenous drug abuse (20–53%) or hemophilia patients (48–80%).[16]

Groups with an intermediate risk in the U.S. are those in whom HBV is acquired through sexual transmission. Sexual acquisition of delta is much less efficient than for hepatitis B. In homosexual men with chronic HBsAg who deny IVDA, the prevalence ranges from 10%–23%.[10, 16] Among female prostitutes from different areas in the United

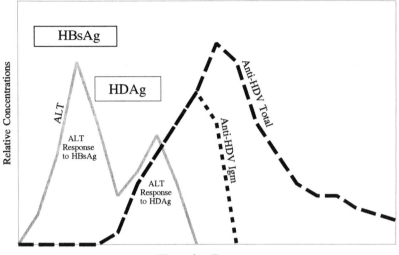

Figure 13.2 A typical serological course of acute resolving delta coinfection based on references 3, 4, 6, 7, 12. HDAg is only detected for 7–21 days. IgM anti-delta persists for two months. Total anti-HDV lasts one to two years.

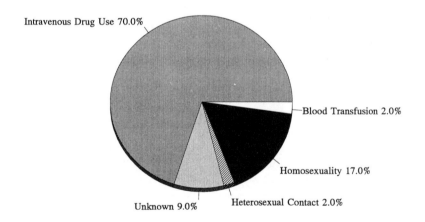

Figure 13.3 Sources of infection for delta virus. Data derived from DeCock KM, et al. Delta hepatitis in the Los Angeles area: A report of 126 cases. *Ann Intern Med* 1986; 105: 108–114.

States, the prevalence of HDV in HBV carriers ranges from 6%, in those denying IVDA, to 21% among those admitting IVDA.[17]

HDV is virtually undetectable among Alaskan natives or Canadian (Inuit) Eskimos who acquire HBV infection perinatally or during childhood.[16]

Relative to worldwide endemicity, Hadler and Fields defined four broad classifications of HDV infection: (*i*) *very low* prevalence when HDV is present in less than 2% of asymptomatic HBV carriers; (*ii*) *low endemicity* when 3–9% of HBV carriers are coinfected with HDV; (*iii*) *moderate endemicity* when prevalence is 10–19% in asymptomatic HBV carriers; and (*iv*) *high endemicity* when HDV occurs in more than 20% of asymptomatic HBV carriers.[4] The worldwide distribution of HDV infection is shown in Figure 13.4. The distribution of HBV for comparison is shown in Figure 7.3.

Notable discordance between the prevalence of HBV and HDV occurs in the Orient. The prevalence of chronic HBsAg carriers is very high among the general population and ranges from 5% to more than 20%. In contrast, HDV prevalence is very low (<2% asymptomatic HBV carriers).

Another peculiar geographical variation in delta disease occurs in South America. In the Amazon basin and among certain Indian groups in Venezuela and Columbia, the prevalence of delta infection is the highest in the world.[6] In one study, 100% of chronic hepatitis B cases were coinfected with delta virus. Fulminant hepatitis is common in this area and appears exclusively due to coinfection or superinfection with HBV and HDV.[18] This disease has been known since 1934 as *Labrea hepatitis* (black fever) and is a rapidly progressive hepatitis with death in one to two weeks. Histopathology shows microvesicular fat infiltration and eosinophilic necrosis.[6, 18] This pathologic picture is different from the standard histiologic picture of severe hepatitis seen with delta in other areas.[9] Risk factors for acquiring HDV infection in this area appear to be sexual transmission among young adults or living in a household with a person with acute HDV infection.[19] Open skin lesions due to impetigo, scabies or dermatoses are thought to be a risk factor for transmission in young children.[19]

Body fluids such as saliva, breast milk, stool, semen and vaginal secretions have not been tested for the presence of delta. Since sexual transmission occurs, semen and vaginal secretions may be presumed to be infectious. The potential for saliva to be a potential vehicle for transmission is unknown. However, there is no reason to suspect that disease transmission pathways that are absent in HBV—fecal-oral, water borne, or airborne—occur for HDV.[4]

Natural History

Chronic delta hepatitis is a more serious and progressive disease than either chronic hepatitis B alone or chronic hepatitis C. Early studies suggested the development of cirrhosis in chronically infected delta patients to be as high as 60–70% versus 15–25% in hepatitis B or C.[7] While delta hepatitis is still felt to be the most severe form of viral hepatitis, the natural history is much more variable than previously thought.

For reasons unknown, geographical location or ethnic background affects the severity of disease. In northern Europe, the U. S. and Italy, over 90% of cases result in liver disease; while in Rhodes, Greece and the Samoan Islands in the Pacific Ocean, the majority of HDV-infected subjects are asymptomatic and healthy.[20]

As in hepatitis C, all natural history studies have had a selection bias in that only patients with chronic liver disease have been followed.[6] Only one population based study among 216 Yucpa HBV carriers in Venezuela has been performed. A five year follow-up of HDV negative HBsAg carriers showed none with moderate or severe liver disease versus 55% of HDV patients who developed moderate or severe liver disease, including 25% who died. A small proportion of each group (1.8%/year) resolved the HBV carrier state.[19]

More evidence which supports the concept that HDV causes severe disease is that the age-prevalence of patients with HDV cirrhosis peaks in the fourth decade of life; that is, one to two decades earlier than the peak age prevalence in HBV or HCV cirrhosis.[20]

Chronic delta infection often causes juvenile cirrhosis. In 26 Italian children, six (26%) presented with cirrhosis.[21] This is in sharp contrast to hepatitis B where cirrhosis is extremely rare in children (see Chapter 6). Fortunately, in the group of 26 children, a 5–12 year follow-up showed a very stable disease picture and no mortality.[21]

Prevention

Hepatitis B vaccine reliably prevents hepatitis B infection, also delta infection since this partial virus needs the helper function of HBV.

Chronic carriers of HBV need to be counseled against behaviors which can lead to superinfection with HDV. Needless to say, in adults, they are often the same behaviors (IVDA, promiscuous sexual activity, etc.) that led to the HBV infection in the first place.

In closed institutions, such as prisons, efforts should be made to keep inmates with HDV segregated from chronic carriers of HBsAg.[22]

Nosocomial transmission of delta hepatitis to other chronic HBsAg carriers on renal hemodialysis has been documented. Carriers of delta hepatitis should therefore be dialyzed on separate machines from patients who are HBsAg positive and delta negative.[23]

Conceivably a vaccine could be made to protect chronic carriers of HBsAg from delta infection. Little work has been done on such a vaccine. In animal studies, some degree of prevention and certainly amelioration of disease due to HDV has been seen.[24]

Treatment

Treatment with alfa-interferon

Early trials of alfa-interferon for disease caused by HDV were disappointing. Doses of 3–5 million units (MU) thrice weekly led to improvements in aminotransferases 25–42% of the time but relapse uniformly occurred after cessation of therapy.[25]

Farci et al. completed a trial of higher dose alfa-interferon in 41 patients given 3 MU and 9 MU three times weekly for 12 months. Serum aminotransferases fell to normal in 70% (9 MU) and 28% (3 MU). With a two to three year follow-up, 50% of those given the highest dose had a sustained remission of ALT values compared to none of the patients given the lower dose. However, HDV-RNA reappeared in all patients after therapy.[26]

The Kings College group in London treated 11 patients with a tapering 12 month dose starting at 10 MU daily and ending at 3 MU three times weekly. Only six patients completed 11 months of therapy but 4 lost HBsAg and experienced improvement or normalization in biochemical parameters. The dropouts were noteworthy: three patients felt self-injection stressful and resumed illicit drugs and two cirrhotic patients developed severe thrombocytopenia causing therapy to be stopped.[27]

Alfa-interferon is not approved for treatment of delta hepatitis in the United States. Given the poor prognosis, a trial of therapy seems advisable by a liver specialist interested in alfa-interferon therapy. Details of monitoring and selection are the same as for hepatitis B and are reviewed in Chapter 8.

Dr Hoofnagle at the National Institutes of Health has suggested therapy be started at doses of 5 MU daily or 9–10 MU three times weekly. If there is no improvement in alanine aminotransferase values (ALT) in three months, alfa-interferon should be stopped. If ALT levels improve, therapy should be continued for at least twelve months. If HBsAg becomes negative, a sustained response can be expected. If HBsAg remains present, therapy should probably be stopped even though a relapse is likely.[25]

Liver transplantation

Fulminant hepatitis and end-stage liver disease due to chronic HDV/HBV infections are two clinical situations in which liver transplantation may be considered.

Fulminant hepatitis is ten times more common in acute delta infection than with any other hepatitis agent. Mortality rates for acute liver failure due to HDV have varied considerably. A large world-wide study shows a 53% mortality rate in fulminant hepatitis secondary to acute HBV/HDV co-infection and a 72% mortality rate in HBsAg superinfection with HDV.[28] In other words, 28 to 47% of patients will survive without transplantation, depending on the mode of infection. There is a 55% development of HDV chronicity in those who survive fulminant hepatitis.[28] Similar survival rates are reported in Los Angeles. In the latter study, when age-stratification was done, no survivors over age 40 were noted.[29]

In a large European multicenter study, the five year survival of patients transplanted for *fulminant* HDV infection was 70%. In the 30% who died, almost all did so within three months of transplantation. The five year recurrence of HDV infection in the allograft in this group was noted to be 40%.[30] In the same trial, the five year survival of patients transplanted for *cirrhosis* due to HDV was 88%. The recurrence rate of HDV infection in the allograft transplanted for cirrhosis due to HDV was 32%.[30]

The major problem for transplanting hepatitis B is recurrence of disease and accelerated cirrhosis and appearance of hepatocellular carcinoma. This subject is reviewed in chapter six. For uncertain reasons, the frequency of recurrent accelerated disease when HDV/HBV is transplanted is much less than for hepatitis B alone. Again, the large European trial showed death from recurrent disease on an average of twelve months in 15.4% of 201 HBV transplants versus 2.7% of 110 patients transplanted for HDV-related cirrhosis.[30] The lower incidence of HDV reinfection of the transplanted liver, and possibly the lower rate of accelerated disease, is probably related to the lower rate of HBV replication caused by the delta virus.[31]

Special Topics

Pediatrics

The natural history of HDV in children is reviewed earlier in the chapter. HDV is essentially the only hepatitis virus to commonly cause juvenile cirrhosis but this pathological outcome is not inevitable even if chronic active hepatitis is present. Most children either present with antibody to the hepatitis B "e" antigen (anti-Hbe) or develop this antibody on 5–12 year follow-up.[14] The presence of anti-Hbe connotes a marked diminution in HBV viral replication and this probably explains the stability of the clinical picture of HDV in this age group.

Treatment with high dose alfa-interferon (5 MU thrice weekly) in 12 children did not produce any sustained remissions; however, three of four HBeAg positive children converted to anti-Hbe during therapy.[14]

Pregnancy

A well nourished woman with delta hepatitis occurring during pregnancy fares no worse than if she were non-pregnant.[32] As in hepatitis B, no increased incidence of fetal malformations are noted.

Limited data suggests that perinatal transmission of delta hepatitis rarely occurs. Seven mothers (one with HBeAg and six with anti-Hbe) were positive for anti-HD out of a tested pool of 6,111 women in Italy. The six babies born to the anti-Hbe mothers remained negative for HBV markers and anti-HD disappeared at three months of life. The baby born to the HBeAg mother developed HBsAg and increasing titers of anti-HD at six months of age consistent with chronic delta infection.[33]

Human immunodeficiency virus (HIV)

In Western countries where HDV infection is acquired parenterally or sexually, a significant number of patients are also infected with HIV. This was emphasized in our unit where a young man with aggressive delta infection was placed into apparent disease remission after high dose alfa-interferon (8 MU daily) therapy only to subsequently acquire HIV infection.

In homosexual patients with anti-HD antibodies, half of whom were also IVDA, 96% were also infected with HIV.[34] In New York, 35% of chronic HBsAg carriers are infected with both HDV and HIV.[35]

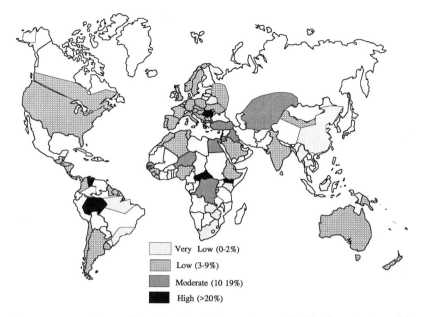

Figure 13.5 Prevalence of hepatitis D in HBsAg carriers worldwide. Figure in the public domain.

HIV infection appears to lessen the liver disease associated with chronic hepatitis B infection; in contrast, the increased severity of liver disease associated with HDV infection appears to be maintained in the presence of HIV-infection.[35] Death in a 30 month follow-up often occurred in patients with triple infection.[36]

There are no reports of alfa-interferon for treatment of HBV/HDV and HIV infection.

Medical Advice for Acute and Chronic Delta Infection

1. The medical advice for patients with acute delta infection (coinfection or superinfection of a chronic HBsAg carrier) is the same as for acute hepatitis B (Chapter 4). More vigilance for the possibility of fulminant hepatitis is needed since this occurs ten times more commonly in delta infection.
2. The advice for chronic delta infection is the same as for chronic hepatitis B (Chapter 5). In Western countries, warnings about continued behavior which led to HDV infection can also cause HIV infection cannot be overemphasized.

3. Alfa-interferon treatment and liver transplantation is available for selected patients.

References

1. Purcell RH. The discovery of the hepatitis viruses. *Gastroenterology* 1993; 104:955–963.
2. Diener TO. Hepatitis delta virus-like agents: an overview. In: Hadziyannis SJ, Taylor JM, Bonino F, eds. *Hepatitis Delta Virus Molecular Biology, Pathogenesis, and Clinical Aspects.* New York: Wiley-Liss, 1993: 109–115.
3. Rizzetto M. The delta agent. *Hepatology* 1983; 5:729–737.
4. Hadler SC, Fields HA. Hepatitis delta virus. In: Belshe RB, ed. *Textbook of human virology.* St Louis: Mosby-Yearbook, 1991: 749–766.
5. Rizzetto M. Hepatitis delta virus. Presentation at American Association of Liver Disease. 1986; Chicago, Illinois. Material in syllabus. (Published by SLACK, Inc., Thorofare, NJ).
6. Polish LB, Gallagher M, Fields HA, et al. Delta hepatitis: molecular biology and clinical and epidemiological features. *Clin Microbiology Review* 1993; 6:211–229.
7. Hoofnagle JH. Delta hepatitis and the hepattis delta virus. In: Seeff LB, Lewis JH. *Current Perspectives in Hepatology.* New York: Plenum, 1989: 47–62.
8. Rizzetto M, Bonino F, Verme G. Hepatitis delta virus infection of the liver: progress in virology, pathobiology, and diagnosis. *Sem Liver Disease* 1988; 8:350–355.
9. Purcell RH, Gerin JL. Hepatitis delta virus. In: Hollinger FB, Robinson WS, Purcell RH, et al., eds. *Viral Hepatitis.* New York: Raven Press, 1991: 175–187.
10. DeCock KM, Govindarajan S, Chin KP, et al. Delta hepatitis in the Los Angeles area: a report of 126 cases. *Ann Intern Med* 1986; 105:108–114.
11. Raimondo G, Craxi A, Longo G, et al. Delta infection in hepatocellular carcinoma positive for hepatitis B surface antigen. *Ann Intern Med* 1984; 101:343–344.
12. Salassa B, Daziano E, Bonino F, et al. Serological diagnosis of hepatitis B and delta virus coinfection. *J Hepatol* 1991; 12:10–13.
13. Aragona M, Macagno S, Caredda F, et al. Serological response to the hepatitis delta virus in hepatitis D. *Lancet* 1987; 1:478–480.

14. Rizzetto M. Hepatitis delta virus: biology and infection. In: Shikata T, Purcell RH, Uchida T, eds. *Viral Hepatitis C, D and E*. New York: Excerpta Medica, 1991: 327–333.

15. Rector WG, Govindarajan S, Penley KA, et al. Delta hepatitis in Denver. *West J Med* 1988; 149:40–42.

16. Alter MJ, Hadler SC. Delta hepatitis and infection in North America. In: Hadziyannis SJ, Taylor JM, Bonino F, eds. *Hepatitis Delta Viru Molecular Biology, Pathogenesis, and Clinical Aspects*. New York: Wiley-Liss, 1993:243–250.

17. Rosenblum L, Darrow W, Witte J, et al. Sexual practices in the transmission of hepatitis B virus and prevalence of hepatitis delta virus infection in female prostitutes in the United States. *JAMA* 1992; 267:2477–2481.

18. Bensabath G, Hadler SC, Soares P, et al. Hepatitis delta virus infection and labrea hepatitis. *JAMA* 1987: 258:479–483.

19. Hadler SC, De Monzon MA, Rivero D, et al. Epidemiology and long-term consequences of hepatitis delta virus infection in the Yucpa Indians of Venezuela. *Am J Epidemiol* 1992; 136:1507–1516.

20. Rizzetto M. Hepatitis delta virus disease: an overview. In: Hadziyannis SJ, Taylor JM, Bonino F, eds. *Hepatitis Delta Virus: Molecular Biology, Pathogenesis, and Clinical Aspects*. New York: Wiley-Liss, 1993:425–430.

21. Bortolotti F, DiMarco V, Vajro P, et al. Long-term evolution of chronic delta hepatitis in children. *J Peds* 1993; 122:736–38.

22. Bader TF. Hepatitis B in prisons. *Biomed Pharmacother* 1986; 40:248–251.

23. Lettau LA, Alfred HJ, Glew RH, et al. Nosocomial transmission of delta hepatitis. *Ann Intern Med* 1986; 104:631–635.

24. Ponzetto A, Eckart M, D'Urso N, et al. Towards a vaccine for the prevention of hepatitis delta virus superinfection in HBV carriers. In: Hadzigannis SJ, Taylor JM, Bonino F, eds. *Hepatitis Delta Virus Molecular Biology, Pathogenesis, and Clinical Aspects*. New York: Wiley-Liss, 1993:207–210.

25. Hoofnagle JH, DiBisceglie AM. Therapy of chronic delta hepatitis: an overview. In: Hadziyannis SJ, Taylor JM, Bonino F, eds. *Hepatitis Delta Virus: Molecular Biology, Pathogenesis, and Clinical Aspects*. New York: Wiley-Liss, 1993:337–343.

26. Farci P, Mandas A, Coiana A, et al. Treatment of chronic hepatitis D with interferon alfa-2a. *N Engl J Med* 1994; 330:88–94.

27. Lau JY, King R, Tibbs CJ, et al. Loss of HBsAg with interferon-therapy in chronic hepatitis D virus infection. *J Med Virology* 1993; 39:292–296.

28. Saracco G, Macagno S, Rosina F, et al. Serologic markers with fulminant hepatitis in persons positive for hepatitis B surface antigen. *Ann Intern Med* 1988; 108:380–383.

29. Govindarajan S, Chin KP, Redeker AG, et al. Fulminant B viral hepatitis: role of delta agent. *Gastroenterology* 1984; 86:1417–1420.

30. Samuel D, Muller R, Alexander G, et al. Liver transplantation in European patients with the hepatitis B surface antigen. *N Engl J Med* 1993; 329:1842–1847.

31. Tur-Kaspa R, Ilan Y, Eid A. Liver transplantation for patients with hepatitis delta infection. In: Hadziyannis SJ, Taylor JM, Bonino F, eds. *Hepatitis Delta Virus: Molecular Biology, Pathogenesis and Clinical Aspects.* New York: Wiley-Liss, 1993; 389–391.

32. Mishra L, Seeff LB. Viral hepatitis, A through E, complicating pregnancy. *Gastro Clinics North America* 1992; 21:873-887.

33. Zanetti AR, Ferroni P, Magliano EM, et al. Perinatal transmission of the hepatitis B virus and of the HBV-associated delta agent from mothers to offspring in northern Italy. *J Med Virol* 1982; 9:139–148.

34. Solomon R, Kaslow R, Phair J, et al. Human immunodeficiency virus and hepatitis delta virus in homosexual men. *Ann Intern Med* 1988; 108:51–54.

35. Novick DM, Farci P, Croxson TS, et al. Hepatitis D virus and human immunodeficiency virus antibodies in parenteral drug abusers who are hepatitis B surface antigen positive. *J Infect Dis* 1988; 158:795–803.

36. Housset C, Pol S, Carnot F, et al. Interactions between human immunodeficiency virus-1, hepatitis delta virus and hepatitis B virus infections in 260 chronic carriers of hepatitis B virus. *Hepatology* 1992; 15:578–583.

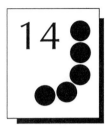

Hepatitis E

History

Since the availability of serology for hepatitis A and B in the 1970's, two very different types of non-A, non-B hepatitis became obvious: a percutaneous form, hepatitis C, and one which was spread by fecally contaminated drinking water. The latter virus has been known as enterically transmitted non-A, non-B virus until 1987 when Robert Purcell of the NIH first proposed the description of hepatitis E for the virus (HEV).[1]

HEV does not cause chronic liver disease. The clinical picture in many aspects resembles the disease caused by hepatitis A. HEV is also an RNA virus but it is in a different family of RNA viruses, *calicivirus*, than the picornavirus family containing hepatitis A.

The geographical distribution, or endemicity, is much more limited for this hepatitis virus than any of the other known hepatitides (Figure 14.1). HEV is apparently not endemic in the United States, Canada, or

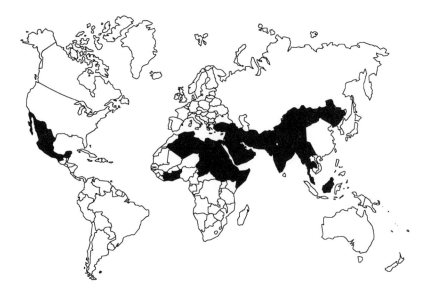

Figure 14.1 Geographic distribution of hepatitis E. The Middle East has been darkened entirely, but cases have only been reported in Turkey, Egypt, Jordan and Kuwait.

other developed countries. It has been reported predominantly in the Indian subcontinent, southern Asian republics of the former USSR, southeast Asia, north Africa and Mexico.

The relevance of understanding this infection for physicians practicing in the United States is that travelers or immigrants can present with a non-A, non-B, non-C hepatitis illness.

The first report of a U. S. citizen who traveled to an endemic area and manifested symptoms four weeks after arriving home illustrates this problem:

> A 38-year old woman from Denver traveled to Rosarito Beach, Mexico (15 miles south of Tiajuana), for one day only, on February 23, 1991. She had ice with four margaritas at two different restaurants. She also ate salsa and chips. She had no underlying medical problems and reported no excessive alcohol consumption, blood transfusions, or intravenous drug use. She had no history of contact with anyone known to have had hepatitis in the six months before her trip....

On March 17, she had symptoms of headache and nausea. She became jaundiced on March 23, at which time her serum aspartate aminotransferase level was 2100 IU per liter, her alkaline phosphatase level 516 IU per liter, and her total bilirubin level 4 mg/dl (127 %μmol/L). Physical examination was normal except for jaundice. Markers for infections with hepatitis A, B, and C were negative, and ultrasonography of the liver was normal. Her symptoms and jaundice resolved by April 17. The fluorescent-antibody blocking assay for antibody to hepatitis E virus was positive in serum samples obtained in April 18 and May 31, with titers of 1:512 and 1:128, respectively. This assay detects antibodies that react with the recombinant C2 structural protein of the hepatitis E virus. Serum antibodies to the same protein were also detected in a Western blot assay.[2]

The vehicle of transmission in this case is probably the ice consumed with the four margaritas at two different restaurants.

In Mexico, epidemics of hepatitis E infection have occurred in Huitzililla and Telixtac, rural villages 70 miles south of Mexico City.[3]

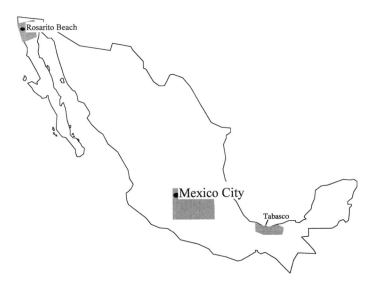

Figure 14.2 Areas in Mexico where acute cases or surveillance for HEV has been done.

The worrisome aspect of the above case is that the source of infection was 15 miles south of the United States border.[4] U. S. travelers to other endemic areas and immigrants have acquired HEV.[5,6] Mexico appears to be the only country in the Western Hemisphere to have HEV as an endemic infection. Figure 14.2 shows those areas of Mexico where cases or surveillance has been reported. In Tabasco, Mexico, the general population has a 6% seroprevalence of HEV by an enzyme immunoassay method from Abbott.[7]

Diagnosis

Early identification of HEV was done by discovery of virus-like particles, which measured from 27 to 34 nm, in stool (Figure 14.3). Visualization of the virus in stool is difficult due to the low levels excreted and the labile nature of HEV in storage.[8]

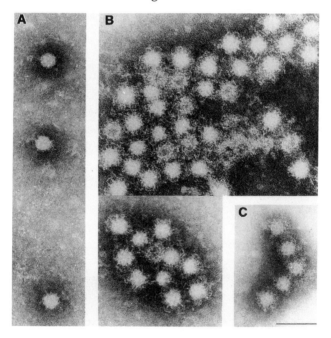

Figure 14.3 Hepatitis E virus in the bile collected on day 30 from a cynomolgus monkey inoculated on day 0 with HCV. **A** Three virus particles without antibody. **B** Upper, immune complex containing 60 particles; lower, complex of 11 particles; both with high antibody rating. **C** Complex of 5 particles with high degree of antibody presence (bar=100 nm). Ticehurst J, et al. Infection of Owl Monkeys and Cynomolgus Monkeys with hepatitis E virus from Mexico. *J Infect Dis* 1992; 165:835–45. Photo courtesy of Dr. John Ticehurst. Photo in Public Domain.

FA Blocking Assay for Anti HEVAg

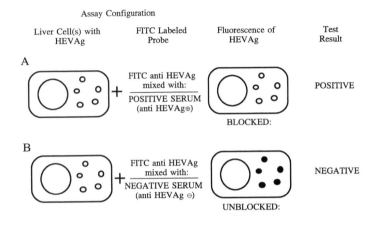

Figure 14.4 Schematic representation of the fluorescent antibody blocking test. Used with permission from K. Krawczynski. Figure in Public Domain.

Immune election microscopy (IEM) has been the only reliable means of identifying both HEV antigen and antibody.[8] The fluorescent antibody blocking test (FABT) (Figure 14.4) was developed from experimentally infected non-human primates.[9] IEM, while very specific, is a cumbersome test; however, all new immunoassays should be validated with it.[8] IEM has shown that geographically distinct viral isolates are cross reactive with each other suggesting one virus or a class of serologically related viruses is responsible for HEV infection worldwide.[10]

Recombinant HEV proteins from epidemic isolates have been verified with FABT and are used in anti-HEV immunoassays such as immunoblotting (Western Blot) or enzyme immunoassay (EIA).[10]

Western Blot IgG antibodies were detected in 93% of patients with active hepatitis thought due to HEV. The continuous presence of IgG anti-HEV was found in 90% of cases over a 24 month observation period. IgM antibodies were detected in 73% of patients within 26 days after onset of jaundice, in 50% one to four months after onset, in 6% six to seven months later and in none after eight months.[11]

EIA, with four recombinant HEV proteins, has been used to look at 45 patients from an epidemic in Kashmir. 71% of patients were positive for IgG anti-HEV; of these, 75% were positive for IgM anti-HEV.[10]

EIA testing of different global populations has given repeatedly positive EIA samples ranging from 2.3 to 15%.[10] Anti-HEV was detected in 2.1% of randomly selected American blood donors.[12] The significance of EIA positivity in blood donors in a non-endemic area remains unclear. Travel to endemic regions, cross-reactive antibodies or infection with nonpathogenic HEV strains have not been ruled out.

HEV-RNA by polymerase chain reaction has recently been developed. Profiles of HEV-RNA occurrence in stools and serum are not yet established.[10]

The role of HEV in fulminant hepatitis (FH) occurring in non-endemic areas also needs clarification. Six of twenty patients with FH in Philadelphia, Pennsylvania (USA), thought due to either non-A, non-B hepatitis (15) or drug toxicity (5), tested positive for immunoblot antibodies or HEV-RNA.[13] Five of 30 patients in a London study of fulminant hepatitis also had evidence of HEV-RNA in sera but none in liver tissue.[14] A subsequent report on these latter five patients showed two to be immigrants from the Indian sub-continent and the other three were British tourists who had recently traveled to Northern Africa.[15] Thus, there appears to be little evidence that HEV causes fulminant hepatitis in non-endemic areas.

Clinical Features

Table 14.1 lists symptoms and signs associated with an epidemic of HEV. Children less than age 14 and subjects older than fifty seldom exhibit jaundice or other symptoms of clinical manifestation.[3,1] Chil-

Table 14.1 Symptoms and signs of hepatitis E in adults. Data derived from references 20,30.

Symptoms	%
Anorexia	70
Nausea	90
Malaise	95
Vomiting	50
Signs	**%**
Hepatomegaly	81
Splenomegaly	25
Jaundice	90
Fever	40
Arthralgia	17

dren, as in all other types of viral hepatitis, are much more prone to have a subclinical presentation.[16] There are no clinical features which separate HEV infection from any other type of viral hepatitis.

The incubation period ranges from two to nine weeks with a mean of six weeks.[1] Laboratory findings in a volunteer are noted in Figure 14.5. Total serum bilirubin in one epidemic was noted to be 4.8 ± 4.5 mg/dl (163 ± 153 µmol/L) in 155 subjects.[18] 8% of patients can develop prolonged jaundice lasting for more than one month associated with light-colored stool and itching. In patients above age 55, the incidence of prolonged jaundice may be as high as 42%.[19]

A significant difference between hepatitis A and HEV is the case fatality rate (CFR). The CFR of hospitalized hepatitis A patients is 1-2 per 1,000 compared to epidemics of HEV where the overall CFR has been 1–2% or more.[1] The cause of death is usually fulminant hepatitis.

A striking difference between HEV and all other types of viral hepatitis is the CFR in pregnant women (Table 14.2).[19, 20] For hepatitis types A, B, C, D, the pregnant woman fares no differently than her non-pregnant counterpart. The CFR increases throughout pregnancy and is worse in the third trimester. In addition to fulminant hepatitis, pregnant women develop an atypical form of diffuse intravascular

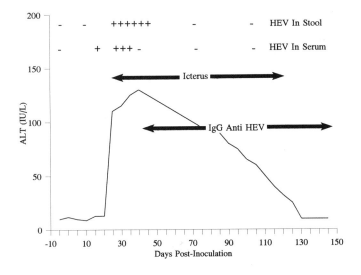

Figure 14.5 Laboratory findings in a volunteer with HEV infection. Used with permission Chauhan A, et al. Hepatitis E transmission to a volunteer. Volume 341:149-150 © by *The Lancet Ltd.*, 1993.

Table 14.2 Case fatality rate for pregnant women in epidemics of HEV in Nepal and China. The nonpregnant female CFR was 0.18% in the Nepal outbreak (data derived from references 19,20).

Stage	Nepal (%)	China (%)
First Trimester	0	1.5
Second Trimester	16.6	8.5
Third Trimester	32.4	21

coagulation. Caesarean section does not appear to improve the outcome.[21]

Fortunately, no evidence exists to suggest that hepatitis E progresses to a chronic infection.[22] When liver tissue has been examined in epidemics, about 50% of cases have a *cholestatic* pattern and 50% a "standard" viral hepatitis pattern. These patterns return to normal histology when the clinical infection resolves. Massive hepatic necrosis has been observed in fatal cases.[10]

The variation of clinical disease as subclinical cases in children, acute icteric illness in young adults, fulminant hepatitis in advanced pregnancy and prolonged cholestasis in the elderly indicate that the outcome of HEV infection is probably dependent on host immunity rather than the dose or virulence of the virus.[19]

Epidemiology—Sporadic vs Endemic

Hepatitis E infection occurs in the setting of epidemics and sporadic cases in endemic areas. Cases which occur in non-endemic areas are imported by travel. Contaminated water appears to be the principal vector of infection. Specific food contamination has not been identified.[3, 24] Prior to serological identification, the clearest understanding came from outbreaks with a compressed curve of incidence or more prolonged epidemics with multiple peaks of cases. The source of the disease in both patterns is usually contaminated water as epidemics are frequently observed following the rainy season.[3, 10] The virus appears to be susceptible to a water pH of less than 3.5.[24]

Epidemics have involved large numbers of cases. 29,000 cases occurred in New Delhi, India in 1955 and 1956. These were shown retrospectively using stored sera to be non-A, non-B in 1980[23] and more recently to be HEV antibody positive.[25] In northwest China (Uighar region), 119,280 clinical cases were observed from 1986 to 1988.[20]

Retrospective serological testing of 17 major non A, non B epidemics in India since 1955 shows that 16 were due to HEV.[25] The secondary attack rate of HEV among exposed household members is low but higher than among non-exposed households (7.7 vs 1.3 per 1,000 population in a Rangoon outbreak). The low secondary attack rate is unusual for enterically transmitted agents and may be due to the relative instability of HEV.[10]

Sporadic cases, independent of an epidemic, are less predictably due to HEV. A retrospective analysis of 75 acute non-A, non-B hepatitis cases in India revealed that 34 had IgM HEV antibodies by immunoblot, 9 with HCV-RNA present and 32 which tested negative for all viral hepatitis serology. 25 of the 75 samples were tested for cytomegalovirus (CMV) and all 25 were negative. CMV is an unlikely cause of adult viral hepatitis in India since 98% of the population has antibodies by age 15.[26]

A third of acute non-A, non-B, non-C cases in Hong Kong appear to be due to hepatitis E.[27] 6% of acute hepatitis A cases also had IgM HEV by EIA making it possible to have coinfection occur. Both hepatitis A and E can be transmitted by infected water making a double infection possible.[27]

Detection of HEV in serum of a presymptomatic volunteer patient by polymerase chain reaction for a few days makes parenteral transmission theoretically possible but unlikely as in HAV infection.[17]

No evidence has been found for heterosexual transmission.[18] Since feces are infected, transmission with homosexual practices, as in hepatitis A, will likely occur but have not yet been reported.

Prevention

A report from India has shown that prophylactic gammaglobulin manufactured from a local source in India proved to decrease, but not at a statistically significant level, the number of cases and severity of disease when compared to the control group.[28] In prophylactic trials performed in Nepal and Mandalay with gammaglobulin prepared from Western countries, no protection was noted.[29] Given the extremely low antibody prevalence rate in Western countries, it would be expected that gammaglobulin derived from non-endemic areas would not be protective.

The issue is very important for pregnant women during epidemics and further work needs to be done in the area of gammaglobulin prophylaxis for HEV.

Summary

Hepatitis E causes a clinical disease very similar to acute hepatitis A. HEV virus appears to be much less stable than HAV and this may account for the low secondary attack rate noted during epidemics. HEV has a limited geographical distribution and cases in non-endemic areas are imported by travelers or immigrants. Contaminated water is the best understood vector of transmission. An unusual feature of HEV disease is the striking fatality rate in pregnant women where as many as 20% can succumb.

In non-endemic areas, serological testing should only be pursued in patients who have had a travel history in the prior three months. In the United States, testing is available from the Centers for Disease Control.

Hepatitis E Outline

1. The clinical sign traditionally used as a marker for disease due to hepatitis E has been jaundice. Anicteric cases occur but are currently poorly understood.
2. Transmission occurs through contaminated water.
3. Hepatitis E causes a clinical picture of benign disease very similar to one caused by hepatitis A. Hepatitis E does not develop into a chronic carrier state.
4. In contrast to other types of viral hepatitis, pregnant women, particularly in the third trimester, can suffer fatality rates as high as 32%.
5. Testing of hepatitis E should only be done in non-A, non-B, non-C viral hepatitis cases which have been in endemic areas.
6. General treatment measures as outlined in Chapter 1

References

1. Purcell RH, Ticehurst JR. Enterically transmitted non-A, non-B hepatitis: epidemiology and clinical characteristics. In: Zuckerman AJ, ed. *Viral Hepatitis and Liver Disease*. New York: Alan Liss, 1988: 131–137.
2. Bader TF, Polish LB, Krawczynski K, et al. Hepatitis E in a U. S. traveler to Mexico. *N Engl J Med* 1991; 325:1659.
3. Velazquez O, Stetler HC, Avila C, et al. Epidemic transmission of enterically transmitted non-A, non-B hepatitis in Mexico, 1986-1987. *JAMA* 1990; 263:3281–3285.

4. Clark C. Dangerous form of hepatitis traced to Baja. *San Diego Union* (newspaper). Dec 5, 1991; page B-1.
5. Centers for Disease Control. Hepatitis E among U. S. travelers, 1989-1992. *JAMA* 1993; 269:845–846.
6. DeCock KM, Bradley D, Sandford NL, et al. Epidemic non-A, non-B hepatitis in patients from Pakistan. *Ann Int Med* 1987; 106:227–230.
7. Ramos-Diaz M, de Medina M, Hutto C, et al. Serological survey for hepatitis E virus among pediatric health care providers in Tabasco, Mexico. *Hepatology* 1993; 18:77 (abstract).
8. Ticehurst J. Identification and characterization of hepatitis E virus. In: Hollinger FB, Lemon SM, Margolis HS, eds. *Viral Hepatitis and Liver Disease*. Baltimore: Williams and Wilkins, 1991: 501–513.
9. Krawczynski K, Bradley DW. Enterically transmitted non-A, non-B hepatitis: identficiation of virus-associated antigen in experimentally infected Cynomolgus macaques. *J Inf Dis* 1989; 159:1042–1049.
10. Krawczynski K. Hepatitis E. *Hepatology* 1993; 17:932-41.
11. Favorov MO, Fields HA, Purdy MA, et al. Serologic identification of hepatitis E virus infections in epidemic and endemic settings. *J Med Virol* 1992; 36:246–250.
12. Dawson GJ, Chan KH, Cabal CM, et al. Solid-phase enzyme-linked immunosorbant assay for hepatitis E virus IgG and IgM antibodies utilizing recombinant antigens and synthetic peptides. *J Virol Methods* 1992; 38:175–186.
13. Munoz SJ, Bradley DW, Martin P, et al. Hepatitis E virus found in patients with apparent fulminant non-A, non-B hepatitis. *Hepatology* 1992; 16:76A (abstract).
14. Sallie R, Tibbs C, Silva AE, et al. Detection of hepatitis E but not C in sera of patients with fulminant NANB hepatitis. *Hepatology* 1991; 14:68A (abstract).
15. Kuwada SK, Patel VM, Hollinger FB, et al. Non-A, non-B fulminant hepatitis is also non-E and non-C. *Am J Gastroenterology* 1994; 89:57–61.
16. Goldsmith R, Yarbough PO, Reyes GR, et al. Enzyme-linked immunosorbent assay for diagnosis of acute sporadic hepatitis E in Egyptian children. *Lancet* 1992; 339:328–330.
17. Chauhan A, Jameel S, Dilawari JB, et al. Hepatitis E virus transmission to a volunteer. *Lancet* 1993; 341:149–150.
18. Khuroo MS, Duermeyer W, Zargar S, et al. Acute sporadic non-A, non-B hepatitis in India. *Am J Epidemiol* 1983; 118:360–364.
19. Shrestha SM, Enteric non-A, non-B hepatitis in Nepal: clinical and epidemiological observations. In: Shikata T, Purcell RH, Uchida T,

eds. *Viral Hepatitis C, D and E*. New York: Excerpta Medica, 1991: 265–275.

20. Zhuang H, Cao XY, Wang GM. Enterically transmitted non-A, non-B hepatitis in China. In: Shikata T, Purcell RH, Uchida T, eds. *Viral Hepatitis C, D and E*. New York: Excerpta Medica, 1991: 265–275.

21. This comment came from a discussion for which I cannot recall the person making the comment. I would like to give proper credit for the communication.

22. Khuroo MS, Saleem M, Ramzan Teli M, et al. Failure to detect chronic liver disease after epidemic non-A, non-B hepatitis. *Lancet* 1980; 2:97–98.

23. Wong DC, Purcell RH, Sreenivasan MA, et al. Epidemic and endemic hepatitis in India: evidence for a non-A, non-B hepatitis virus etiology. *Lancet* 1980; 2:876–878.

24. Jothikumar N, Aparna K, Kamatchiammal S, et al. Detection of hepatitis E virus in raw and treated wastewater with the polymerase chain reaction. *Applied and Environmental Microbiology* 1993; 59: 2558–2562.

25. Arankalle VA, Chadha MS, Tsarev S, et al. Serologic evidence fo a second epidemic non-A, non-B hepatitis agent. *Hepatology* 1993; 18:77 (abstract).

26. Arankalle VA, Choke LP, Chadha MS, et al. Aetiology of acute sporadic non-A, non-B viral hepatitis in India. *J Med Virology* 1993; 40:121–125.

27. Lok AS, Kwan WK, Moeckli R, et al. Seroepidemiological survey of hepatitis E in Hong Kong by recombinant-based enzyme immunoassays. *Lancet* 1992; 340:1205–1208.

28. Joshi YK, Babu S, Sarin S, et al. Immunoprophylaxis of epidemic non-A, non-B hepatitis. *Indian J Med Res* 1985; 81:18–19.

29. Purcell RH, Shikata T. General discussion [on hepatitis E]. In: Shikata T, Purcell RH, Uchida T, eds. *Viral Hepatitis C, D and E*. New York: Excerpta Medica, 1991: 379–387.

30. Xue-Yi C, Xue-Zhong M, Yu-Zhang L, et al. Epidemiological and etiological studies on enterically transmitted non-A, non-B hepatitis in the south part of Xinjiang. In: Shikata T, Purcell RH, Uchida T, eds. *Viral Hepatitis C, D and E*. New York: Excerpta Medica, 1991: 297–312.

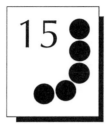

Fulminant Hepatic Failure

Evaluation
Survival Probability
Special Problems

Fulminant hepatic failure (FHF) or fulminant hepatitis is defined as altered mental status (i.e., hepatic encephalopathy) and coagulopathy occurring within eight weeks of the onset of symptoms referable to the liver in those previously well.[1, 2]

The list of causes for FHF is long,[1] but in practical terms, viral hepatitis and drug-induced injury account for the vast majority of cases. In reported series, the most common cause of FHF is acute viral hepatitis, accounting for up to 72 percent of all cases.[2] The proportions of viral agents are noted in Figure 15.1. Non-A, non-B viruses appear to be the most common cause in the United States; of this group, hepatitis C appears to account for only a minority of cases.[3, 4, 5] Hepatitis E is not a cause of FHF in the United States.[6]

While viral hepatitis is the most common cause of fulminant hepatitis, any given case of viral hepatitis rarely progresses to FHF. The incidence of FHF in all types of acute viral hepatitis is much less than one percent. The only exception to this rule occurs in acute delta hepatitis where FHF occurs in 5% or more of cases.

The focus of this chapter will be to help the physician recognize the severity of the liver failure, the probability of survival and when to

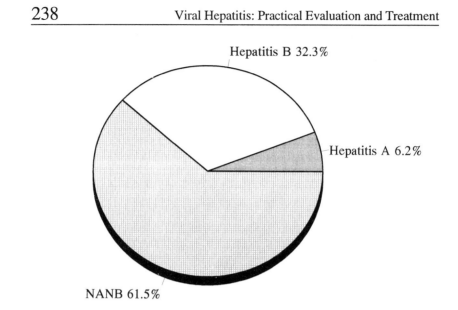

Hepatitis B 32.3%

Hepatitis A 6.2%

NANB 61.5%

Figure 15.1 The proportion of viruses causing fulminant hepatitis in the United States. Compiled from references 3,4. Very few of the NANB cases are caused by hepatitis C.

refer patients for specialized treatment and possible liver transplantation.

Evaluation

Encephalopathy, by definition, is the essential clinical feature of FHF and is graded on a scale of 0 to 4 (Table 15.1).[7] Mental status changes may precede the onset of jaundice. One of the earliest signs is a change in personality with anti-social or uncooperative behavior occurring. Nightmares, headaches and delirium can take place.[8] Later, the picture may include seizures or decerebrate rigidity with spasticity, extension and hyperpronation of the arms.

The grade of encephalopathy determines prognosis since cases that do not progress beyond grade 2, irrespective of cause, have an excellent prognosis. When grade 3 or 4 encephalopathy develops, however, the outcome becomes less predictable.[7] Patients with decerebrate rigidity, loss of the oculo-vestibular reflex and respiratory failure rarely survive.[9]

Severe coagulation changes are typical of FHF since the liver synthesizes all coagulation factors except factor VIII. Bleeding is found in 73% of cases and can be severe in 30%.[10] The most common site is gastroin-

Table 15.1   Clinical features of encephalopathy by grade.

Grade	Clinical Features
1	Mild or episodic drowsiness; impaired ability to perform computations; irritability and tremor may be present
2	Increased drowsiness with confusion and disorientation; rousable and conversant; ataxia usually present
3	Very drowsy and disoriented; obeys simple commands; often agitated and aggressive
4	Responds to painful stimuli at best, but may be unresponsive; signs of cerebral edema may be present

testinal, mainly from gastric mucosal erosions, and the incidence of this complication can be reduced by the prophylactic use of H_2 antagonists.[11] Hemorrhage most often correlates with a low platelet count, particularly under 50,000 per cubic millimeter.[2] Platelets in this condition also do not function properly and exhibit abnormalities in aggregation and adhesion.[10]

As discussed below, the prothrombin time is a very good prognostic indicator. The French have promoted the use of factor V levels for use in prognosis, particularly in acute hepatitis B.[12] In the author's experience, the delayed reporting time from the laboratory for factor V activity makes it an impractical parameter.

Survival Probability

Survival of FHF depends on etiology, age of the patient and clinical parameters such as encephalopathy and certain biochemical and co-agulation parameters.

The most comprehensive experience in FHF comes from the Liver Failure Unit at King's College Hospital in London. Their studies demonstrate a gradual improvement in survival over the past 20 years with medical management alone. The improvement is due to a greater understanding for the role of intensive care in acute liver failure rather than any specific mode of therapy. While overall survival was only 20% in 1973, it has improved to over 50% by 1988, at least for certain groups, such as those with FHF due to hepatitis A or B. Thus, fulminant hepatitis A patients have a much better prognosis (~70%) of survival than fulminant hepatitis B (50%); while non-A, non-B patients fare significantly worse with a 30% survival.[13]

Age affects outcome. Age greater than forty and less than ten are strong predictors of non-survival.[12, 14]

The degree of encephalopathy usually predicts survival with medical or surgical management. The overall survival for those reaching grade III or IV encephalopathy with medical management is 20%. For those with grade I or II encephalopathy, survival is 66%.[8]

Worse results with transplantation were seen in two large series when stage IV encephalopathy was transplanted with survival figures of 28 to 30%. Other series, however, have found no correlation between the grade of encephalopathy being transplanted and outcome.[7]

King's College has developed a model to select patients with FHF for liver transplantation (Table 15.2).[7, 14, 15] A Japanese group tested a number of models and concluded the King's College criterion to be the most sensitive and specific.[16]

The primary prognostic factor in cases not associated with acetaminophen poisoning is the prothrombin time. The King's College group initially reported that a prothrombin time > 100 seconds alone predicts a need for transplantation. However, laboratories in the United Kingdom use human brain derived thromboplastin which differs substantially from the rabbit brain derived thromboplastin used in the United States. This variation in reporting has led to recommendation that international normalized ratios (INR) be used.[15] The prothrombin times in Table 15.2 have been changed from the original values to the updated INR ratios of 6.7 and 4.7.[7] In addition, Table 15.2 lists age parameters, duration and degree of jaundice and non-A, non-B etiology as parameters for consideration of liver transplantation.

Table 15.2 Model used at King's College to select patients with fulminant hepatic failure for liver transplantation (Acetaminophen overdose parameters excluded). Used with permission. O'Grady JG, et al. Fulminant Hepatic Failure. In: Schiff L, Schiff ER, eds. *Diseases of the Liver.* Philadelphia: JB Lippincott, 1993; 1086.

Prothrombin time, INR > 6.7
or
Any three of the following:
Unfavorable cause (non-A, non-B hepatitis, or drug reaction)
Jaundice > 7 days before encephalopathy
Age < 10 or > 40 years
Prothrombin time INR > 4.7
Serum bilirubin > 300 μmol/L (17.6 mg/dl)

What should the practicing physician away from a liver transplantation unit do with a case of FHF? Using the parameters listed here, the possibility of survival without transplantation can be balanced with a decision for transplantation referral.

If the patient with hepatitis A can survive FHF without transplantation, the liver regains normal functioning without fibrosis. The long-term outcome after recovery of FHF due to hepatitis B is variable. Karvountis et al.[18] found only one of 16 patients who were initially HBsAg positive to remain so after about two years of follow-up. HBsAg detection was by a less-sensitive counterelectrophoresis method commonly employed in the early 1970's. Galambos, et al., followed nine survivors long-term after FHF due to hepatitis B : five had normal histology (2 HBsAg⁻, 3 HBsAg⁺), one had portal inflammation (HBsAg⁻), and three had chronic active hepatitis or cirrhosis.[19] Long-term follow-up of survivors with medical management having non-A, non-B fulminant hepatitis has not been reported.

The decision for liver transplantation is not inconsequential. Receiving an orthotopic liver commits a patient to life-long immunosuppression with its attendant side-effects and monitoring (including periodic liver biopsies). A higher primary allograft non-function may occur when transplanting for FHF (33%) as compared to chronic disease patients (5–10%); this is thought due to factors released from the native necrotic liver.[1] In addition, reinfection may recur in hepatitis B, C and D.[17] The problems of transplantation need to be highlighted; otherwise, patients think that receiving a new liver is like having a new part placed in their car whereby they can drive away without any further worries.

If doubt exists about the suitability of transplantation, contacting the nearest center by telephone and discussing the case is appropriate.

It is beyond the scope of this chapter to review in detail the clinical care of patients with FHF. Excellent mechanics of care are discussed in several reviews.[1, 2, 20] However, several salient points will be highlighted.

Special Problems

Infection

Bacterial and fungal infections are common in FHF.[2] In fact, sepsis unrelated to the liver may mimic FHF and the possibility of this problem should be aggressively pursued upon presentation. The

King's College group reported four cases which were transferred to the Liver Failure Unit only to be diagnosed with sepsis rather than FHF.[21]

Daily cultures of all types should be obtained with aggressive antibiotic therapy. Prophylactic antibiotic regimens have not shown any benefit.[22]

A search for herpes simplex viral hepatitis should be made in pregnant and immunocompromised patients in FHF since administration of acyclovir may be life saving in these situations.[23,24]

Hypoglycemia

Low blood glucose levels result from defective gluconeogenesis in the liver. Hypoglycemia may alter mentation in some patients and blood glucose levels should be monitored closely and 10 or 20% glucose solution given. A 20% glucose solution given during transport of the patient to another medical center is recommended.[8]

Bleeding

Bleeding commonly occurs from gastric mucosal lesions. A reduction in bleeding from this source with prophylactic H^2 blockers has been demonstrated.[11] Attempts to correct hemostatic defects with fresh frozen plasma and platelets are indicated only if bleeding occurs or prior to invasive procedures.[25]

Hepatic encephalopathy

The precise etiology of hepatic encephalopathy (HE) is uncertain; however, secondary factors may precipitate its appearance. These factors include gastrointestinal hemorrhage, electrolyte disturbances, sedatives, infection, hypoglycemia and hypoxemia.[25]

Cerebral edema is an ominous finding and early signs are systolic hypertension, increased limb muscle tone, and sluggish pupillary responses.[2,25] Management of cerebral edema should be undertaken by those experienced in its treatment.

Lactulose is often recommended but there is no proof of its benefit in FHF. It is difficult to administer lactulose when patients are in grade III or IV encephalopathy.[7] The mechanisms for HE in acute liver failure and chronic liver failure may be quite different.

Conclusion

Every physician needs to understand and evaluate for the rare possibility of fulminant hepatic failure occurring during acute viral hepatitis. The responsibility of the non-specialist is to monitor early findings and triage the care of such patients.

References

1. Fingerote RJ, Bain VG. Fulminant hepatic failure. *Am J Gastroenterology* 1993; 88:1000–1010.
2. Lee WM. Acute liver failure. *N Engl J Med* 1993; 329:1862–1872.
3. Emond JC, Aran PP, Whittington PF, et al. Liver transplantation in the management of fulminant hepatic failure. *Gastroenterology* 1989; 96:1583–1588.
4. Lidofsky SD, Bass NM, Prager MC, et al. Intracranial pressure monitoring for fulminant hepatic failure. *Hepatology* 1992; 16:1–7.
5. Wright TL. Etiology of fulminant hepatic failure: is another virus involved? *Gastroenterology* 1993; 104:640–653.
6. Kuwada SK, Patel VM, Hollinger FB, et al. Non-A, non-B fulminant hepatitis is also non-E and non-C. *Am J Gastroenterology* 1994; 89:57–61.
7. O'Grady JG, Portman B, Williams R. Fulminant hepatic failure. In: Schiff L, Schiff ER, eds. *Diseases of the Liver*. Philadelphia: JB Lippincott, 1993: 1077–1090.
8. Fulminant hepatic failure. In: Sherlock S, Dooley J, eds. *Diseases of the Liver and Biliary System*. London: Blackwell Scientific, 1993: 102–113.
9. Hanid MA, Silk DB, Williams R. Prognostic value of the oculovestibular reflex in fulminant hepatic failure. *BMJ* 1978; 1:1029.
10. O'Grady JG, Langley PG, Isola LM, et al. Congulopathy of fulminant hepatic failure. *Sem Liver Dis* 1986; 6:159–162.
11. Mac Dougal BR, Bailey RJ, Williams R. H$_2$-receptor antagonists and antacids in the prevention of acute gastrointestinal hemorrhage in fulminant hepatic failure. *Lancet* 1977: 1:617–619.
12. Bernuau J, Goudeau A, Poynard T, et al. Mulivariate analysis of prognostic factors in fulminant hepatitis B. *Hepatology* 1986; 6:648-51.
13. Hughes RD, Wendon J, Gimson AE. Acute liver failure. *Gut* (suppl) 1991:S86–91.
14. O'Grady JG, Alexander GJ, Hayllar KM, et al. Early indicators of prognosis in fulminant hepatic failure. *Gastroenterology* 1989;97:439–445.

15. Munoz SJ, O'Grady JG, Hambley H, et al. Prothrombin time in fulminant hepatic failure. *Gastroenterology* 1991; 100:1480–1481.
16. Watanabe A, Shiota T, Tsuji T. Prognostic assessment of fulminant hepatitis from indication criteria for liver transplantation. *J Medicine* 1992; 23:39–49.
17. Samuel D, Muller R, Alexander G, et al. Liver transplantation in European patients with the hepatitis B surface antigen. *N Engl J Med* 1993; 329:1842–1848.
18. Karvountzis GG, Redeker AG, Peters RL. Long-term follow-up studies of patients surviving fulminant viral hepatitis. *Gastroenterology* 1974; 67:870–877.
19. Horney JT, Galambos JT. The liver during and after fulminant hepatitis. *Gastroenterology* 1977; 73:639–645.
20. Lidofsky SD. Liver transplantation for fulminant hepatic failure. *Gastroenterology Clinics of North America* 1993; 22:257–268.
21. Dirix LY, Polson RJ, Richardson A, et al. Primary sepsis presenting as fulminant hepatic failure. *Q J Med* 1989; 73:1037–1043.
22. Rolando N, Gimson A, Wade J, et al. Prospective controlled trial of selected parenteral and enteral anti-microbial regimen in fulminant liver failure. *Hepatology* 1993; 17:196–201.
23. Klein NA, Mabic WC, Shaver DC, et al. Herpes Simplex virus hepatitis in pregnancy. *Gastroenterology* 1991; 100:239–244.
24. Kusne S, Schwartz M, Breining MK, et al. Herpes simplex virus hepatitis after solid organ transplantation in adults. *J Infect Dis* 1990; 163:1001–1007.
25. Martin P, Maddrey WC. Fulminant hepatic failure. *Practical Gastroenterology* 1990; 14:50–59.

Index

REQUIRED READING FOR THE FAMILY PHYSICIAN

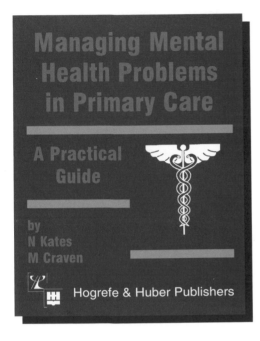

1997 / 384 pages / hardcover / ISBN 0-88937-124-5 **$49.00**

"This is a book that addresses the foundations of good mental health care in family practice and represents a breakthrough in practical use for family physicians struggling with the burden of care of most mental health problems in our communities."

Walter Rossen, Professor and Chair
Department of Family and Community Medicine
University of Toronto, Canada

"There is clear "how to do it" advice, rather than having treatment described in theoretical terms..."

David Goldberg, MD
Director of Training and Research
Institute of Psychiatry
London, UK

This very practical handbook is designed to help family physicians increase their skills in both identifying and managing a wide range of mental health problems in their patients. The authors emphasize effective, time-saving strategies for the busy doctor, and include numerous interviewing and management tips as well as advice on involving families, utilizing community resources, and making appropriate referrals.

"Drs Kates and Craven have written an eminently practical and useful text for family physicians and family practice residents.... Clearly the authors bring a perspective from real world practice experience. Family physicians must acquire the knowledge and skills to recognize and manage patients' psychological problems."

R Schneeweiss, MD
Professor and Chair
Dept of Family Medicine
University of Washington, Seattle

To order please mail or fax the completed coupon to:
H & H Publishers, Seattle Main Office,
PO Box 2487, Kirkland, WA 98083-2487, USA
Phone (206) 820-1500, Fax (206) 823-8324

Call toll-free [800] 228-3749

Order Form

[ ] Check enclosed.   [ ] Please bill me.
[ ] Charge my: [ ] VISA   [ ] MC   [ ] AmEx

Card # _____

Exp date _____ Signature _____

Shipping address (please include phone & fax)

I would like to order	US$	Qty	Total
Schutte: ...*Medical Malpractice Suits*	129.00		
Kates: *Managing Mental Health...*	49.00		
Subtotal			
Shipping & handling: $4 for the first book; $1 for each add'l book			
WA residents add 8.2% sales tax			
Total			

"... [This course] ... teaches doctors how to avoid creating the grounds for most malpractice suits... This isn't an instruction manual about how to cover up negligence or incompetence. It's ... intended to help good, competent practitioners recognize and avoid the lapses in communication and record-keeping that underlie most preventable malpractice suits."

From Melvin Belli's Foreword

Preventing Medical Malpractice Suits shows physicians, dentists, nurse practitioners, clinical psychologists, and their support staff how to protect themselves from threats of potentially damaging legal actions through the application of a few rules, practical aids, and checklists which a practitioner can use immediately.

*"**Today's physicians need this information**... Dr Schutte captures the impact of the lawsuit experience from the perspective of the physician defendant...*

*It's plain talk for a **population of professionals** who can bank on being targeted in a matter of litigation in their fututre, maybe more than once.*

*From the perspective of the **staff worker or office nurse**, the author explains a sophisticated view of prevention, and the true value to a physician of a committed and vigilant support staff... the real risk managers, in my opinion.*

*Plain talk. Definitely should also be used in **teaching institutions for emerging physicians.**"*

Ellen Hughes, Risk Manager
Midwest Group, Kaiser Health Centers

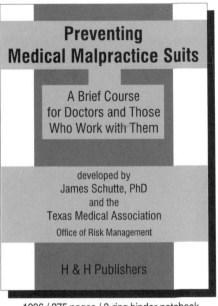

Preventing Medical Malpractice Suits

A Brief Course
for Doctors and Those
Who Work with Them

developed by
James Schutte, PhD
and the
Texas Medical Association
Office of Risk Management

H & H Publishers

1996 / 275 pages / 3-ring binder notebook
$129.00
[not for distribution in Texas]

The Benefits –

We invite you to utilize this effective home study material, developed in close cooperation with the Texas Medical Association:

• The American Academy of Family Physicians has approved this course for 12 credits of prescribed continuing education.

• It contains highly practical information which you can use in your daily practice.

• Your malpractice insurance carrier may offer lower rates as a result of your having completed this brief course; please check with your particular agent.

• Very down-to-earth material, smoothly presented by professional medical writers. Also very interesting to patients.

• This information is highly relevant for *all* members of your staff.

This [material] attempts to explain how to avoid medical malpractice suits and does it in a clear and concise manner. The advice is aimed at physicians as well as the entire office team including nurses, managers, and other health care personnel.

This ... is a must for all physicians practicing medicine** and surgery in order to reduce risks of malpractice claims. It is clearly written, and covers all aspects of physician-patient relationship, office personnel, care in the hospital, billing, and medical records. **I recommend this [material] without reservation to be read completely and to be followed in all aspects.

Melvin A Shiffman, MD, JD, Tustin, CA,
in *American Journal of Cosmetic Surgery*,
Vol. 13, No. 1, March 1996.